...rge class

...mon mental health ...that is extensively used in Britain and internationally. He is now Director of Stress Control Ltd.

He is a Fellow of the British Psychological Society, a Fellow of the British Association for Behavioural and Cognitive Psychotherapies, a Chartered Psychologist and Chartered Scientist.

Stress Control

Jim White

ROBINSON

ROBINSON

First published in Great Britain in 2017 by Robinson

1 3 5 7 9 10 8 6 4 2

A CIP catalogue record for this book
is available from the British Library.

Important note
This book is not intended as a substitute for medical advice or treatment.
Any person with a condition requiring medical attention should consult a
qualified medical practitioner or suitable therapist.

ISBN: 978-1-47213-710-4

Typeset in Gentium Basic by Hewer Text UK Ltd, Edinburgh
Printed and bound in Great Britain by CPI Group (UK), Croydon CR0 4YY

Papers used by Robinson are from well-managed forests and other responsible sources.

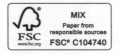

Robinson
An imprint of
Little, Brown Book Group
Carmelite House
50 Victoria Embankment
London EC4Y 0DZ

An Hachette UK Company
www.hachette.co.uk

www.littlebrown.co.uk

For Lilian, Kirsty, David and Neil

Contents

1

How this book works

Introduction

Stress is part and parcel of life. We all get it. Think of blood pressure: if you are alive, you have blood pressure. If you are alive, you have stress. If your blood pressure gets too high, you should do something about it; it's the same with stress. This book aims to help you do just that.

Stress, for most people, is a mix of anxiety, depression, feelings of panic, poor sleep, low self-confidence, low self-esteem and a poor sense of well-being. It is one of the most common problems in the world today.

It is easy to feel overwhelmed by stress, and even the idea of reading a book about it can be daunting. To make the process as easy as possible the use of jargon has been avoided, and straightforward language used throughout.

This book aims to teach you to become your own therapist. It offers a five-step plan to control your stress:

Step 1 Know your enemy – learn about stress and how it affects you.

Step 2 First steps – straightforward ideas to give an instant sense of control.

Step 3 Fight back – linked skills for long-term control of stress.

Step 4 Boost your well-being – skills to improve your life.

Step 5 Stay on top of your stress – skills to control your future.

This approach combines cognitive-behavioural therapy, positive psychology and mindfulness. There are no easy answers, no miracle cures. But with hard work and practice, you *can* learn to control your stress.

The five steps are made up of a range of skills. These skills can best be seen as parts of a jigsaw – each is important on its own, but it is only when all the pieces are slotted together that the bigger picture can emerge.

Let's look at these steps in greater detail:

Step 1 Know your enemy

Before you can fight back against your stress you have to understand it. So the first step is to learn about stress and how it affects you. **Chapter 2** looks at what stress is, describes the most common signs and examines what causes it and keeps it going. It looks at the 'what ifs' of anxiety and the 'if onlys' of depression. It looks at how stress affects your feelings, your thoughts, your body and the way you act. We'll see who gets it and how common it is. We will look at the vicious circle of stress to explain why, once it gets a grip, it keeps hold. Using this knowledge we can then build a positive circle to weaken that grip. These vicious and positive circles will act as maps that will guide you throughout the book and show the progress you are making.

I will describe the Mind, Body, Life model and how the skills taught in the book link to this. There is much to be said for the 'healthy body, healthy mind' principle so we'll look at a range of skills to boost both. These will be combined with well-being skills aimed at improving your life. While it is always good to reduce feelings of stress, this in itself does not always lead to *feeling* better. Some people just feel *empty* rather than *well*. By learning ways to boost well-being we can be surer of being less stressed *and* feeling better.

Chapter 3 takes this a step further. You can use your knowledge of what stress is to learn a lot more about *your own* stress – to know your enemy. No two people feel stress in exactly the same way, so we need to work out why *you* suffer it in the way you do. This introduces the 'becoming your own therapist' role as you start to identify your own patterns, which then helps you to work out the best ways to control your own stress. You might want to go through these with someone close to you whose views you trust. They might see things you don't. If your views differ, try to work out why this is and learn from it.

This detailed self-assessment breaks into five stages:

1 **Describe your stress** Eleven questions looking at the past, present and future. This lays the foundation for the remaining stages.

2 **Work out the patterns** Nine questions to take this one step further. Why are you stressed at some times but not others? Why in some places and not others? You should learn a lot about your stress here. In itself, this can start to reduce that stress.

3 **Life inventory** The following eight areas look at stress mainly from the 'Life' part of the Mind, Body, Life model: your nature, job, health, relationships, money, home/neighbourhood, behaviour and strengths. Too often we only see the bad things – the weaknesses – and so it is vitally important to look at your strengths (things you may pay little attention to). You need this knowledge when you come to boosting your well-being in Chapter 10.

4 **Measure your stress and well-being** Three of the best stress questionnaires can be found in this section. You can complete each, score it and make sense of your score – know where you stand. You can refer to these as you work your way through this book to see what progress is being made.

- The GAD-7 measures anxiety.
- The PHQ-9 measures depression.
- The WEMWBS measures well-being.

5 **Stress Control aims** to weaken the vicious circle that keeps stress alive and bring to life the positive circle that will keep you on top of stress. In this stage, your task is to build your own vicious circle.

6 **Set your goals** Your goals should be based on what you have learned in the other four parts. We look at good and bad goals.

These goals act as your guiding star as you learn the skills offered in the book (but don't be afraid to modify your goals as you learn more).

Step 2 Making a start

Now you know your enemy, **Chapter 4** helps you to get yourself into the best shape and then to pick up some weapons to allow you to fight back.

Sometimes, stress can so overwhelm you that you feel there is no way you can get any control over it. So, at Step 2, we learn straightforward skills that can work well in the short term. This helps you build self-belief as you go on to learn the long-term skills in Step 3. It will help you get rid of the things that may be helping keep stress alive. Then we'll look at some great self-help ideas you can use to build a sense of control. It divides into three:

- Clearing the decks – where you get rid of things that might be keeping stress alive.
- Finding hidden problems – a final check in case you missed anything while clearing the decks.
- Twenty-five ways to cope – run through these, choose the ones that best fit and try them out.

Step 3 Fight back

This is where you will learn the powerful skills that can help you keep control of your stress.

Chapter 5 looks at how the body reacts in the way it does, and explains why. The breathing and relaxation techniques described will help your mind relax as much as your body in the Mind, Body, Life model.

There are five skills in this chapter:

- Limiting caffeine.
- Exercise.
- Belly breathing.
- Progressive relaxation.
- Healthy eating.

In Chapter 6, building on what we learned in Chapter 5, we focus on what, for many people, will be the crucial part of the book. We explain how and why our minds react to stress. We look at the common sense voice versus the stress voice; look at 'grasshopper thinking' and 'the blinkers' and, with this knowledge, move onto the three skills of the chapter:

- Building the foundation.
- The Big 5 Challenges.
- Breaking stress up.

Many people will start to feel the pieces of the jigsaw coming together in **Chapter 7** as they see how the Body and Thought skills merge with the Action skills. We look at how actions are affected by stress and divide them into *avoidance* and *behaviour*. We show how each feeds stress and how, by learning the skills, we can learn to starve the stress. The three skills are:

- Facing your fears.
- Stepping out of your comfort zone.
- Problem solving.

A good number of people have actual panic attacks, but just about all of us have panicky feelings. **Chapter 8** looks at skills to tackle both. One of the big issues with panic is the 'fear of fear' where you become afraid of the way you have reacted to fear, and so fear that something awful is happening to you because, e.g. your heart is racing or you feel breathless. This chapter will look at different types of panic feelings and explain how to cope with them or, even better, how to prevent them. We will look at the role of breathing in some detail. There are four main skills:

- Controlling your body.
- Controlling your thoughts.
- Controlling your actions.
- Reducing the risk of feeling panicky.

Stress often leads to poor sleep; poor sleep leads to stress. In **Chapter 9** we look at why getting a good night's sleep and recharging your batteries is crucial to controlling daytime stress. We will look at the 'sleep cycle', the importance of deep and dream sleep (REM), different types of sleep problems and reasons for poor sleep. There are two sleep skills:

- Sleeping tips.
  - Your sleeping needs.
  - Your bedroom.
  - Calming your body.

        □ Calming your mind.
        □ Building up good habits.
- Retraining your sleep.

Step 4 Boost your well-being

Chapter 10 focuses on all aspects of the Mind, Body, Life model. Up until now we have worked on getting rid of bad things: stressed thoughts, panicky feelings, poor sleep, etc. Now we turn to strengthening good things and, by doing so, boosting your sense of well-being.

We'll look at why well-being is crucial to controlling stress. We'll look at 'flourishers' and 'languishers' and why 'flourishers' do so well in life. We then focus on helping you to 'flourish'. There are three stages:

- Four steps to well-being: connect, be active, keep learning, give.
- Mindfulness: take notice.
- Be the best version of you: compassion and gratitude.

Step 5 Stay on top of your stress

In **Chapter 11** we make sure you can see the big picture and show you how to use your new skills to face the future with confidence. You will learn about SMART goals as a useful way to tackle problems, and will find tips on ways of coping.

Each of the chapters is one piece of the jigsaw which, once put together, will allow you to see the bigger picture that leads to stress control.

The ultimate aim of this book is to turn you into your own therapist. So the final, and most important, piece of the jigsaw can now be slotted into place – you. Believe in yourself. Because *you* matter.

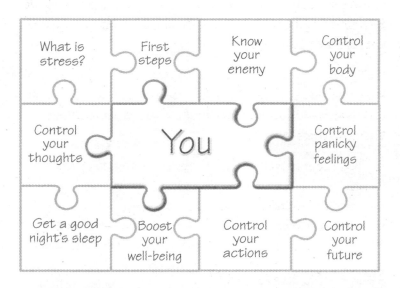

2

What is stress?

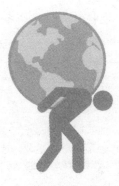

Stress affects us in so many ways and we all react differently to it. The most common form of stress is a mix of *anxiety* (tension, nerves, worry) and *depression* (feeling flat, sad). Most of us will experience anxiety and depression at some time in our lives.

Stress is often associated with sleep problems, loss of confidence and/or self-esteem, feelings of panic and of anger or irritation. You may find yourself drinking too much or relying too much on medication as a way of coping. You may feel your nature has changed for the worse.

Stress

Anxiety

Depression

Anger

Panic

Sleep problems

Low self-confidence and self-esteem

Drinking too much / using drugs

If any one word best describes stress, it is 'overwhelmed' – the feeling that life has just got too much for us. If one image best describes stress, it is the idea that you have the weight of the world on your shoulders. Combine this with the feeling that there is nothing you can do to control it and stress will get a solid grip of you – and will hang on tight.

Stress isn't black and white. We all have stress in our lives, and some times are worse than others. This may be due to what we have to face: work pressures, money problems, ill health, family problems and so on. Yet many people find it hard to work out why they are stressed; those who don't seem to have problems in their lives also get stress. The truth is that we all worry, and we all feel down from time to time. We might not be able to take all the weight off our shoulders but, by learning stress control, we can lighten the load.

Mark

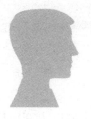

'I should feel great just now. I've got no real problems in my life. Yet I'm pretty flat and don't have any get-up-and-go. Just can't be bothered; my concentration is all over the place and I can get really narky with my girlfriend for no reason and I don't know why.'

Anne

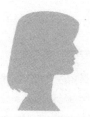

'It's been one thing after another this year. Moving to the new house, all the changes at work, and my daughter has been ill on and off for months. I'm so stressed out and I'm just not coping well with it at all.'

When does stress become a problem?

There are three clear indicators that your stress level is getting too high:

When you can't get rid of it even when you try hard to do so
If you have had a rotten, stressful day at work but come home and manage to switch off by phoning a friend, taking the dog out, listening to music and so on then you have ways to control your stress. If, however, you try again and again to reduce the stress but nothing works, it is time to learn some skills to control it.

When it comes and goes for no reason It's normal to feel stress, e.g. when sitting an exam, after a fall-out with your friend, worrying about paying a bill. But if you are feeling stressed at times when you know you should be relaxed, such as when lying in bed, sitting in front of the TV, having a night out, and so on, then it is time to learn those skills.

When it moves to the centre of your life If your brother phones and suggests meeting up for a drink on Friday and you say, 'Great, but let's wait till nearer the time and I'll see how I feel' then stress is starting to control you. It is time to learn ways to control it.

If you can recognize yourself in these examples you may feel that your mind is being taken over by stress. You might even feel as if you are cracking up. You might feel that you can't cope with things that others seem to cope with (or things you could cope with in the past). If so, you are doing the right thing in using this book.

Stress is not the same as a 'fit of the blues' or 'having an off day'. A good kick up the backside will not shift stress. It is a lot more complex than that. Stress becomes a problem when we feel we can't *control* it. Stress comes about when the pressures on us outweigh our ability to cope, and affect our day-to-day life. Stress is about us feeling *overwhelmed*.

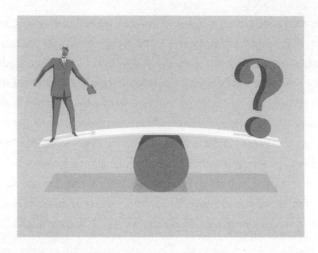

As you will always have pressures and problems in your life, the way to control stress is to learn better coping skills. This shifts the balance in your favour and you are better able to get a grip on it.

Kate is a thirty-eight-year-old office manager, and a single parent of two children. She says she is a born worrier but that over the past three years she has become a 'nervous wreck'.

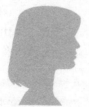

'I worry about daft things: being late for work; what the neighbours think of me; I worry if the kids are five minutes late home from school; just everything. I'm better if I keep myself busy so, oddly, I'm much better at work but I can't relax at all in the house. I never sit at peace for more than five minutes. Though I get to sleep OK I wake up a lot in the night and can't get back to sleep again, turning things over and over in my mind.

'I'm always on edge; I bite the kids' heads off all the time for no reason. I can go for days with a throbbing headache that starts at the back of my neck and goes all the way to the top of my head. I just feel tense all the time. I always feel under threat and think that people are putting me down, even when I really know they're not. I find myself getting into arguments with people in my mind even when there is no need to. I can get so worked up and not know how to calm down again. I might pick over whole conversations to see if I have said or done the wrong thing. I just feel I'm not on top of things the way I should be. I doubt myself all the time, even though my manager says I'm doing great.'

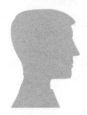

Irfan is forty-seven years old and works as a nurse in a dementia unit. He lives with his wife and three children. He has coped with the usual ups and downs for most of his life and would not normally describe himself as a stressed person. However, after some changes at work, he has started to feel less able to cope.

'I know I am harder to live with and sit in my own world a lot more. I'm not like that so it annoys me that I'm being unfair. I find it much harder to switch off and relax. I can't sit at peace in the house and I drive the family nuts if I've got the remote as I just switch from channel to channel, never watching anything from start to finish. I'm a bit more withdrawn than before – I just can't be bothered doing things I usually enjoy. I love cricket, but now I can't be bothered with it. I worry about daft things that I know I shouldn't worry about. But I can't stop.

'I'm much more aware of my body as well. My heart might speed up a bit, or I might notice my breathing changing. I've been going to the doctor a lot more, worried in case I might be very ill. Sometimes, I can get a bit panicky about this, while there is another part of my mind telling me not to be so stupid. I always seem to feel tired, and I've lost my appetite and have lost a bit of weight. I never feel rested these days. I never feel 100 per cent. To be honest, life seems grey, empty and very hard work, but thinking this makes me feel guilty as I know I have a lot to be thankful for.'

The common signs of stress

Although stress can affect us in a vast number of ways, there are some common signs.

Worry

Often you may find yourself worrying about things that you know you don't need to worry about; or, at least, not to the extent you do. But no matter what you do you can't shut the worries down. A sure sign that stress is getting too high is when you worry *about* worry, e.g. 'Why am I worrying like this? Why can't I get a grip on this? What's wrong with me?'

Lack of energy

Just never feeling 100 per cent. Feeling that you are dragging yourself through the day. You may feel ill or that there is something wrong with you.

Feeling on edge/can't switch off

You may find it hard to relax or feel calm. You might jump for the slightest reason. Oddly, this may be worse at times when you think you should be calm, e.g. sitting in front of the TV, or lying in bed. You might try to keep yourself busy as a way to cope.

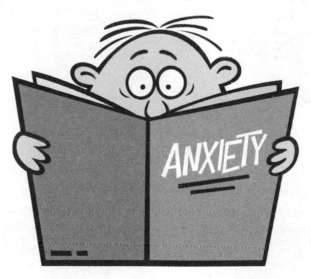

Feeling hopeless

The future appears black and you don't see any way to change it. This means you find it hard to motivate yourself to do things even when you know you should at least try: 'What's the point? Nothing is going to change.'

Waiting for the worst to happen

The *'what ifs'*. You always fear things will work out badly or that you will be unable to cope. This may lead you to avoid doing things or going to certain places. You might find yourself threatened by things your common sense tells you are not really a threat. A fear of being overwhelmed is common here.

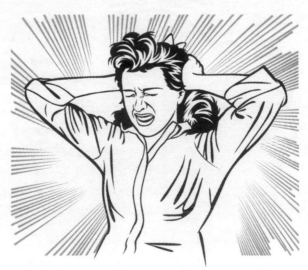

Brooding

The *'if onlys'*. You may find yourself drawn to upsetting things that have happened to you in the past and be unable to stop thinking about them, even though it distresses you. Sadness is often a sign of this. The idea of 'loss' can be important here – feeling that you have lost something of importance in your life. This could be someone close to you dying; losing a good friend; losing a job, and so on. Just like the 'what ifs', these thoughts can go round and round in your head for hours on end.

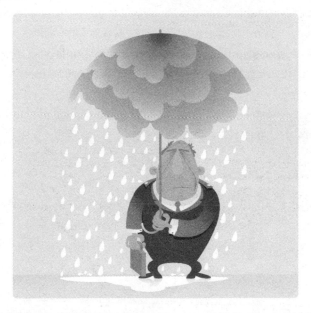

Poor sleep

You may have problems getting to sleep, waking during the night or early in the morning and knowing you will not get back to sleep, so you don't recharge your batteries. Maybe you sleep too much but still don't feel you are rested. All these make you less able to fight off stress the next day (and thus you are less able to sleep the next night, and so on it goes). We will look at the role of vicious circles later on in this chapter.

Feeling irritable/angry

You lose your temper when you know you shouldn't. This often leads to feelings of guilt, and as a result you may become harder to live/work with. So relationships suffer and, as we will see when we look at well-being in Chapter 10, strong relationships help protect us against stress.

Drinking too much

You may drink as a way to relieve your stress, but alcohol often makes it worse (and might make your sleep patterns even more erratic). You may use drugs/medication in the same way.

Avoiding doing things

This could be due to the 'what ifs' – a fear that you won't be able to cope with something you have to do or somewhere you have to go. Or maybe you just let things slip – housework, work or social life. This might be due to lack of energy or 'can't be bothered' feelings. As we will see in Chapter 7, avoidance is one of the most important things keeping stress alive.

Panicky feelings

A sudden feeling that *something* awful is about to happen to you. This often comes with strong physical symptoms: rapid heart rate, fast breathing, sweating, feeling faint. You may fear making a fool of yourself or, at its worst point, that you are having a heart attack, going mad or dying.

Poor concentration

You lose track of conversations, films, books. You may also feel that stress is affecting your memory. You might fear something is going wrong with your brain.

Feeling worthless

Stress rips out your self-confidence and self-esteem. You may feel like a failure and that everyone else is better than you. You never give yourself a break and talk to yourself in ways you would never talk to anyone else. You will avoid challenges and this, of course, just makes things worse.

Tearful/emotional

You may find yourself crying a lot more. Things get to you in ways they would not have done in the past. You may feel you have less control. You might avoid things like the news on TV as you can't cope with watching the more upsetting items.

These are just some of the main ways stress affects us. There are many others, which we will look at in the next section. But if you recognize yourself here then you are doing the right thing – learning ways to get on top of the stress.

The four parts of stress

- **What you feel** The common emotions that make up stress.
- **What you think** What goes through your mind when you are under stress.
- **What you do** How you act when under stress.
- **How your body reacts** Physical symptoms when under stress.

These feed each other to keep stress alive. Let's look at each in turn.

Stress can affect your feelings

You may feel uptight/anxious	You may be very moody or emotional
You may feel flat/depressed or down	You may get jealous easily
You may feel too easily overwhelmed	You may feel physical or emotional discomfort easily
You may feel easily upset	You may feel insecure and vulnerable
You may feel frustrated	You may have lost your sense of humour

You may feel guilty	You may feel life is without hope
You may feel easily embarrassed	You may feel tearful
You may feel low a lot of the time	You may feel that stress brings out the worst in you
You may feel full of anger and resentment	You may become more small-minded, petty and resentful

Stress can affect your thoughts

You may worry or brood about things you know should not bother you	You may find it hard to relax your mind
You may lose self-confidence and self-esteem	You may feel that you can't control your world
You may feel your memory is poor	You may have lost interest in a lot of things
You may feel very self-conscious	You may be easily startled/on edge
You may have a strong fear of rejection	You may not like yourself

You may feel cut off (isolated) from others	You may be waiting for (or expecting) the worst to happen
You may feel you are at the end of your tether	You may feel easily confused
You may find it hard to concentrate even for short periods	You may have a strong fear of failure

Stress can affect your actions

You may avoid doing things or going places as you fear you will not be able to cope with them	You may be drinking, smoking, taking more drugs or relying on medication more than you should
You may be more quick tempered or angry	You may be eating a lot more or a lot less
You may be withdrawing from life, e.g. seeing less of friends and family	You may be more tearful
You may be unable to sit at peace or feel at ease	You may let others walk over you more
You may be making more mistakes at work or at home	You may be impulsive

You may try to 'play safe' more than usual	You may find yourself teeth grinding/jaws clenched
You may try to avoid responsibility	You may stammer

Stress can affect your body

You may have a lot of aches and pains due to tense muscles	You may feel you are dragging yourself through the day
You may be more prone to colds and flu	Your body may feel uptight for much of the day
You may feel drained of energy	You may find that your body reacts very easily to stress, e.g. you get more headaches
You may feel your breathing changes when tense or panicky	You may find it hard to get to sleep; you may wake during the night or early in the morning
You may lose or gain weight	You may have upset stomachs
You may get a lot of headaches	You may have poorer skin

You may never feel 100 per cent	You may suffer palpitations/ increased heart rate
You may sweat more	You may feel dizzy or have surreal feelings

Grace is seventy-four years old. She feels she has had her ups and downs over the years. She has lived alone since her sister died two years ago.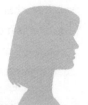

'I suppose I've had a bit of a hard life. My mum died when I was young and I was brought up by my gran who was a very strict lady. There wasn't much love in that house. She always made me feel that I was useless. I grew up very shy and wouldn't say boo to a goose. So I never had that much confidence. But I was lucky to marry George who was a good man and a good provider. We lost our Anne at three months and we took that very hard, and poor George had trouble with drink for a few years after that, but he sorted himself out and we were blessed with three other children. I lost George eleven years ago and, of course, the young ones are all away now – one is in Bristol, one is on the rigs and our youngest boy went off to New Zealand a long time back as there was no work to be had here.

'I moved in with my sister after she lost her husband as money was very tight for the both of us, and we got on just fine and she was good company for me. But she passed on and I'm alone a lot of the time now and I do miss having someone in the house. The days can be long when you're on your own. I'm trying my best to get out and about and I have joined a pensioners' club that gets me out twice a week, and sometimes some of us go out on a Tuesday night for a bite to eat or go to the pictures. But I'm so uptight when I'm out. It's daft, I know. Even though everyone is really nice, I just can't relax. My hands shake – I hate holding out my hand if someone brings me a cup of tea and I'm sure I'll spill it when I put it up to my mouth. If I could get a grip on my nerves, I'd feel so much better.'

Marta is nineteen years old and is out of work just now. She has had panic attacks for the past two years. Her first panic attack was at college; the room was small, hot and full of people. She felt that there was not enough air in the room.

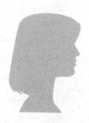

'The panic came on out of the blue. It felt like a cold wave crashing over my head. One minute I was really hot then really cold. My heart was racing and the sweat was pouring off me. I felt as if I was there but not there, if you know what I mean. I was sure I was going to pass out. After that, I was sure that my heart was not right. Even after all the tests came back fine, I still felt I was dying when I had a panic attack. Yet when I feel calm, I know perfectly well that panic attacks won't kill me or make me mad and that they will pass. But this common sense flies out the window as soon as the panic feeling hits me.

'I'm desperate to get a job and not just because I really need the money. I find that I can cope better when I have a good routine. But I'm still tense most of the day. I'm always aware of my heart rate.

'I still find it hard to believe that panic can affect me so badly. I keep asking my flatmates for reassurance about my symptoms and it is beginning to annoy them. Over and above the panic, I'm more tense and down. I think I'm drinking a bit too much as well, and that's not helping.'

Is stress a common problem?

At any point, one in five of us has a stress problem. Not a fit of the blues, not just going through a bad patch, but a real problem that makes us miserable and badly affects our day-to-day lives (and maybe the lives of those close to us too). This same statistic – one in five – is found right across the world. Just under half of us will have a problem with stress at some point in our lives. This makes stress one of the biggest problems we face today. It also looks as if stress is a growing problem globally.

Stress is one of the most common problems dealt with by doctors. We also know that about half of all those with stress do not go to the GP at all, for a variety of reasons. They may not realize that they have it. They may feel that no one can help them. They may feel too ashamed to tell anyone about it. Yet even talking about the stress can help as it may get the sufferer thinking of ways to help themselves.

Is it a 'real' problem?

There is still, for some, a stigma about stress. On the whole people are not keen to admit to it or accept it is stress. Many go to the GP to get help for a physical symptom: headaches, upset stomach, heart racing, and the like. Some feel quite angry if they are told they are suffering from stress.

John

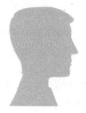

'I told my boss I was stressed out. She just about fell off her seat. She thought I was the most laid-back guy in the place. Yet inside I feel like I'm falling apart.'

Rachel

'A couple of weeks ago, Gerry, my neighbour, asked me what was wrong, said I wasn't my usual self, that I seemed down in the dumps. I just burst into floods of tears. I never do that but it was like the dam bursting inside me and it all came out.'

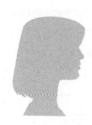

Most people would rather have a 'real' problem like a broken leg. At least you know what caused it, you know how to mend it and you know that, in a few months' time, you will be fine. Stress is not like this. It is often hard to say why you have stress. You may not know what to do to help, and you don't know how you will feel in a few months' time.

Stress is as real as any medical problem. The causes of stress and the things that keep it going are complex. Giving yourself a good shake will do nothing to shift stress. Learning skills to fight back will.

Who gets stress?

All of us. There is nothing 'special' about people who suffer from stress: after all, there are a lot of them. The trouble is that too many people feel they are the only one with the problem, and so feel 'different'. We are good at putting on a mask to hide it. We are then scared that the mask will slip, and this just adds to the stress. So many people may look fine on the outside but feel a mess inside.

Try these questions. The first three are about anxiety, the last two about depression:

Anxiety

Over the last two weeks, have you:

Felt nervous, anxious or on edge?	YES	NO
Found it hard to stop or control worrying?	YES	NO
Have you found yourself avoiding places or activities, and did this cause you problems?	YES	NO

If you answered 'yes' to two out of three *anxiety* may be part of the picture.

Depression

Over the last two weeks, have you:

Often been bothered by feeling down, depressed
or hopeless?   YES   NO

Often been bothered by little interest or pleasure
in doing things?   YES   NO

If you answered 'yes' to two out of two *depression* may be part of
the picture.

Recognize yourself here? Or think you could be going down
that road? If so, you are doing the right thing reading this
book.

Some causes of stress

Many things can cause stress, and Chapter 3 takes a closer look
at the different factors. However, it is often hard to work out
why you have stress. It is often caused by more than one thing,
as explained by looking at the **Mind, Body, Life model**.

We are made up of three main parts:

- **Mind** Our attitudes, the way we think, our beliefs, emotions,
  actions, memories, our coping skills and so on.
- **Body** This can be divided into two: firstly what we are born
  with, e.g. genes and fight/flight systems, and secondly how
  our bodies are affected by illnesses, medications, fitness,
  eating, drinking, smoking and so on.

- **Life** The wider world and how it affects us: family, relationships, wealth/poverty, jobs, unemployment, social life, education and the society we live in.

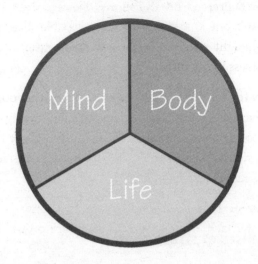

The best way to understand someone is to look at how these three aspects can affect him or her (and how they impact on each other). The more problems in each area, the greater are our chances of having stress. The aim is to understand the things you can control, and recognize and accept what you can't change.

Mind We know that starting life with poor attachments (for example, to our mother) or facing bad events in life can make us more prone to stress. We can't change these facts, but we can learn to challenge the way we think about them; we can learn ways of changing our behaviour and skills to improve our coping strategies. This gets our mind on top form and thus lessens stress and boosts well-being.

Body Some of us are more prone to be worriers; some are more prone to be depressed. But the big word here is *prone*. It doesn't set things in stone. Our brains are more capable of change than we once thought – they can learn, to some extent, to be less prone to stress in the future.

We can try to look after ourselves by ensuring that our body is as healthy as possible. Eating well, exercising, cutting down on caffeine, not drinking too much or using too many drugs all help to lessen stress and boost well-being. This fits well with the idea of 'healthy body, healthy mind'.

Life We know that boring jobs, poor relationships, money concerns and lack of support make us more prone to stress. Some things in life we can't change but, hopefully, some things we can. What we can do is strengthen our contact with others. Too often people feel stress isolates them. This feeds stress. Feeling part of something bigger will always help lessen stress and boost well-being.

This book will look at improving both the Body and Life. But most of the work will focus on the Mind. Think of these three elements as cogs in a gear. If we make one cog move, the others move too. The next pages look at some of the most important factors.

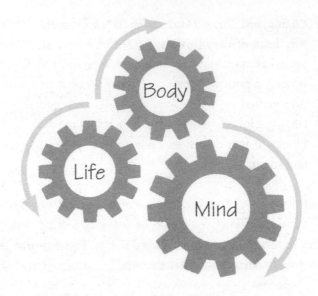

Your nature: childhood

Those people who had a lot of childhood fears (often in the first two years of life) – of the dark, of strangers, of being alone – seem to be more prone to stress in adult life. Children who faced traumatic events in their early years are more prone to stress as adults. Children who took longer to settle at school, who often complained of aches and pains, who were irritable, who were very shy and who found it hard to deal with new situations may also be more prone to stress in later life.

Other childhood factors that make you prone to stress as an adult are:

- Not having a stable, secure and loving upbringing.
- Being 'wrapped in cotton wool' by a parent.

- Coping with stress by avoiding facing problems.
- Any kind of very upsetting event: emotional, physical or sexual abuse; emotional or physical neglect; humiliation.
- Having a family member who had alcohol problems; was imprisoned, or had serious mental health problems.
- Having a lot of changes in your life: moving house, schools, illness in you or others close to you, parents separating, and so on.

Your nature: adulthood

If, by nature, you are easily upset, often tense, prone to low moods or worry, often dissatisfied with yourself and others, or if you feel guilt keenly, then you may be more prone to stress.

Other factors that make you prone to stress as an adult are *life events* – the more changes in life, the more prone most of us become to stress. Good events (birth of a baby, getting a job, moving to a nice area) as well as bad events (death of a parent, losing a job, being mugged) can trigger stress. This is due to having to adjust to change. Too much change in too short a time can result in stress.

Hassles

Many people with stress have a lot of *hassles* in their life. A hassle is a problem that is there day after day. It may be quite small, and it may be hard to do much about it. It may not upset you all that much but slowly it eats away at you. It could be a problem at work, in the home, with the people next door, with debt, coping with illness. These hassles slowly wear you down and stress slowly builds.

Jenna

'It's been one thing after another. We have had a lot of hassle with teenagers hanging about outside. I find myself looking out the window at the slightest bit of noise in the street. My mum is back in hospital and there is talk of lay-offs at work. There is real uncertainty around and I don't like that.'

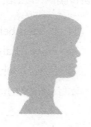

Are women more prone to stress than men?

Most of the books will tell you that women are twice as likely to have stress than men (and therapists tend to see a lot more women than men). However, I think they deal with it in different ways. Due to male pride and stigma, men may be more likely to hide stress and try to deal with it on their own. Women are more likely to seek help from someone like their GP. Men may also drink as a way of coping with stress, and are more likely to have a problem with drink than women. So maybe more men start off with a stress problem, drink to try to control it and end up with a drink problem that is really covering up stress.

May is sixty-one years old. She lives alone and works as a carer. She has been feeling down on and off since she was a teenager. She is concerned that, although she notices when her mood starts to drop, she can't do anything about it.

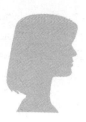

'I go from being fairly happy-go-lucky to feeling I'm weighed down with all the troubles in the world. I know I am hard to work with when I'm like that. Normally, I try to be helpful and pleasant with my workmates and I know they like me. But when I'm like that, although I try to put a face on it, I'm sure I come over as ratty and exasperated over trivial stuff – stuff that I would not normally bother about. My friends have been great but they are fed up with me as I never phone them or go out any more. I know they want to help me but I won't let them get close.

'I can't tell you the last time I felt like having a laugh. I feel a lot more tired than usual, and once I get in from work I tend to slump in front of the TV. I'm deadbeat and just want to sleep all the time. I used to love to read but my concentration is down the tubes. I feel so much guilt at not getting on with it and I wonder if I'll ever feel like my old self again.

'I find when I'm like that I cry more easily – I won't even read the papers these days as there is always something upsetting that I can't handle. My sleep has gone to pot. I don't want to eat – I could do with losing some weight, but not like this. Although some days are better than others, it annoys me that I don't have any way to control my feelings.'

Darren is twenty-six years old. He works in a call centre and lives with his dad. Darren copes well with his job but gets a lot of stress coping with tea breaks.

'If I'm at the table with the guys I work with, I'm OK. If I don't know a lot of them, I go into my shell and I clam up. I find it hard to look at people in the eye. I'm sure they think I'm weird or boring or thick. I find myself working out in advance what I will say and of course that never works out. I can't seem to just talk off the cuff. I think I'll say the wrong thing. I hate signing my name in front of anyone as my hand shakes a lot if I think they are watching me. I'm scared they will say something about it.

'If I'm out with my mate, I tend to drink too much to get a bit of confidence. I know that's not a wise move. There is a woman at work I really like and I want to ask her out on a date, and one of her friends told my mate that she likes me. I screw up my courage but I never go through with it as I know I'll blush like mad and she would just think I'm daft. My confidence has dropped through the floor. No matter where I am, I feel like a fish out of water. I look at all the other guys just being normal while I feel like a failure. Why can't I cope like them?'

Life factors

There is a clear link between stress and what life throws at you. People who live in the poorer areas in our cities are twice as likely to have stress as those in the wealthiest (but, of course, even the richest people can have terrible stress). Other life factors can make people more prone to stress:

- Money problems.

- Being a single parent.

- Lack of control over your life.

- Poorer education.

- Poorer health.

- Lack of support.

- Bad neighbours.

'The house is too cramped for us but we just can't move. My partner has to work all the overtime he can get to keep our heads above water so I don't see him much. I just feel I'm surviving week to week. It's not much of a life.'

'I live in the flats. We've got some real odd people there so I can't let the kids use the lifts on their own. So they're round my feet all day. I've not got the money to take them out a lot. They can drive me mad. School holidays are a killer. My family have their own problems so I don't like to ask them for help. I worry about how I'm going to get by.'

'I'm in a good job, have good friends, but I'm on my own and feel lonely a lot. I have to look after my dad who isn't in the best of health. So, I've got to make sure he is OK – taken his tablets, had something hot to eat, hasn't had a fall and so on. He is a constant worry for me and I don't really like to talk about personal things so I don't have anyone who I can get things off my chest with.'

Common sense tells you that any one of these factors would make any normal person more prone to stress. But they do not tell the whole story. A great many people who do not have any of these problems still suffer from marked stress. At the same time, many people who do have a lot of life problems have low levels of stress.

Something that chimes with some people is the idea of *'low power, excessive demand'*. In other words:

- How much power do you have to control or change your life?
- How many demands are there on you?

The less power and more demand, the more prone you may be to stress. The more power, the more able you should be to control stress.

What we also know is that the kind of society we live in hugely affects stress levels. People living in countries with the greatest gap between rich and poor have much greater levels of stress. And this affects all of us – rich and poor (although it affects the poor more). And the bad news? Britain is one of the most unequal societies in the world. Not much we can do about this (unless we move to Denmark – one of the most equal societies in the world). But, as can be seen from the evidence presented above, it isn't as simple as blaming yourself for having stress – stress affects us for many complex reasons. We can't change them all, but we can focus on the ones we can.

What keeps stress going?

Once stress gets a grip, would you agree with the following statements?

- Self-confidence drops.
- Self-esteem drops.
- You feel threat from all sides.
- You doubt your ability to cope.
- You can't stop your mind racing.
- You start to avoid places or things more.
- Your body reacts more easily to additional stress.
- You may feel your back is to the wall.
- You may feel the stress brings out the worst in you.
- You feel you're losing – or have lost – control of your life . . .
- . . . and you feel overwhelmed with the weight of the world on your shoulders.

Don't worry if you can't see what started your stress as the things that *cause* stress may not be as important as the things that keep it *going*. After stress kicks in, it can change us in all kinds of ways. These changes then often feed the stress and keep it alive.

You will reflect on these changes and feel yourself getting pulled down by them. The sense of control in your life weakens: instead of swimming over the waves, the waves now break over your head and all you can see are bigger waves on the horizon. You may feel it is all you can do to keep your head above the water.

It is only common sense to see that once all these things take hold they will cause your stress to blossom. So, as the causes of your stress fade from the picture, these changes will feed the stress and keep it alive. Put simply, once stress gets a grip of you, it keeps hold. The aim of this book is to teach you how to starve it so that you control stress instead of stress controlling you.

The vicious circle

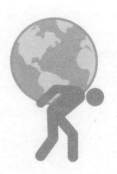

Stress affects so many aspects of our lives: our body, our thoughts, our actions and so on. These form a vicious circle that keeps stress alive. Your stressful thoughts feed your stressed actions. Your stressed actions feed your stressful body. Your stressful body feeds your stressful thoughts. And so on and so on (see the vicious circle below). In Chapter 3 you will draw your own vicious circle. Then, in the following chapters, you will learn the skills to starve this vicious circle, and, in its place, a positive circle will grow.

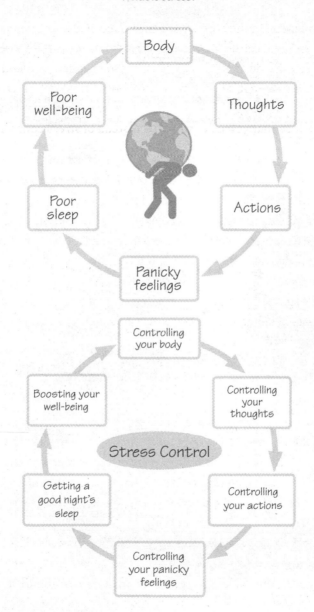

Summary

- Stress is a very common problem. We all have stress. You have too much of a normal emotion – think of it like blood pressure. When it gets too high, we should do something about it. So you should not aim to 'cure' stress but rather to control it.

- Stress usually includes anxiety, depression, anger, feelings of panic or irritability, loss of confidence or self-esteem and poor sleep. Drinking too much, using too many drugs or relying too much on medication are also common.

- The most common signs are: worry, lack of energy, feeling on edge/inability to switch off, drinking too much, feeling hopeless, waiting for the worst to happen, brooding, poor sleep, feeling irritable or angry, avoiding doing things, panic feelings, poor concentration, feeling worthless, feeling tearful/emotional.

- One in five of us is having problems with stress right now. Almost half of us will have a problem with stress at some point in our lives.

- Stress can be caused by a range of things from childhood experiences, life events and everyday hassles to how our societies work. Often, however, it is very hard to see why stress has become such a problem in someone's life.

- Once stress gets a grip of you, it feeds itself by forming a vicious circle.

- Getting stress under control is a lot more complex than just giving yourself a good shake. You need to learn skills to starve the vicious circle and, in its place, build a new positive circle. We do this by combining stress reduction skills with well-being skills to squeeze the stress from both sides. This book gives you the tools to do the job.

- There is no magic cure so try not to be impatient. It will need a lot of hard work on your part. Believe in yourself – it takes time to control stress.

Last words

The aim of Chapter 2 is to help you see what stress is and how it affects people. If you recognize yourself in these pages you are on the right road.

Your next task is to 'know your enemy'. Chapter 3 contains your first major assignment – to assess all aspects of your stress and work out how stress affects you. This will help you work out what your own vicious circle looks like and, using this knowledge, how to starve it.

3

Know your enemy

Before you take aim at the stress, you need to get to know it inside and out. The better you know your enemy, the more able you will be to fight back.

Earlier, I looked at the idea of 'becoming your own therapist'. This chapter starts the ball rolling, and your next step is to work through the following. Give each of them your full attention (it might help to take a break between each stage).

There are six stages:

Stage 1 Describe your stress.

Stage 2 Work out the patterns.

Stage 3 Life inventory.

Stage 4 Measure your stress and well-being.

Stage 5 Draw your vicious circle.

Stage 6 Set your goals.

Stage 1 Describe your stress

Your task now is to get 'under the skin' of your stress and learn how it affects you. The following questions – covering your past, present and future – will help you. Take your time over them. It might help if you write down your answers.

Once you have done this, ask those close to you what they think. Do they agree? Do they see things you don't see? As you go through the book, think about revisiting these questions as you learn more about yourself.

The past

- How long has stress been a problem for you? Has it stayed the same? Has it come and gone? Why is this?
- Do you know what caused the stress initially? Family problems? Life changes? Are you a 'born worrier'?
- Does stress run in the family? If 'yes', why do you think this is?
- What have you tried in the past to help? Did it help? Would it help now?

The present

- How would you describe your stress now?
- How would other people describe your stress? If your views differ, why is this?
- Are there things going on in your life just now which are keeping your stress alive?

- What made you want to tackle your stress now?
- Are you trying anything to help now? Is it working?

The future

- If necessary will you be able to make changes in your life that will help your future?
- How would your life be improved if you had better control of your stress?

Stage 2 Work out the patterns

The next step is to see if you can find a link between your stress level and what is going on in your life at the present time. Think long and hard about these questions and, if you would find it helpful, write down your answers. What do they tell you?

Is there a pattern to your stress? Does it come and go during the day? During the week? During the month? Why is this?

What things make the stress worse? Being out of the house? Being alone? After drinking? Why is this?

What things make it better? Being with the family? Keeping busy? Getting things off your chest? Why is this?

What happens to your body when you are stressed? Heart races? Headaches? No energy? How does this make you feel?

What kinds of things do you worry or brood about when you are stressed? Your job? Your health? Do you feel you are making a fool of yourself? Why is this?

How do you act when you are stressed? Do you avoid doing things? Try to cover up your stress? Shout at others? Why is this?

How do other people know when you are stressed? Ask them.

What parts of your life are most affected by stress? Family life? Work? Why is this?

What parts of your life are least affected by stress? Why is this?

Stage 3 Life inventory

This third stage takes a wider view of what is happening in your life. This broader perspective may help you make more sense of the stress. As before, ask others what they think.

Many areas of life will involve at least some stress. So instead of simple YES/NO questions and answers, you are asked to rate the level of stress in each area using a 10-point scale. The example below looks at how content you are with life:

|-----|-----|-**X**-|-----|-----|-----|-----|-----|-----|

Not at all content   Very content

Note where the cross has been placed. The person is saying that, by and large, he is not very content with his life.

Work your way through the following eight areas by placing a cross at the point that best describes the way you feel. Ignore the areas that do not apply. Stress may *affect* all or most of these areas; but you need to decide whether the stress is under control or if it is adding to your problems. If it is, try to think of ways to control it.

The further to the right you place your cross, the more of a problem it is for you.

Area 1 Your nature

Are you a tense person?

|-----|-----|-----|-----|-----|-----|-----|-----|-----|
Not at all   Very much so

Do you feel down a lot of the time?

|-----|-----|-----|-----|-----|-----|-----|-----|-----|
Not at all   Very much so

Do you feel easily dissatisfied with yourself and others?

|-----|-----|-----|-----|-----|-----|-----|-----|-----|
Not at all   Very much so

Are you easily upset?

|-----|-----|-----|-----|-----|-----|-----|-----|-----|
Not at all   Very much so

Do you easily feel guilt?

|-----|-----|-----|-----|-----|-----|-----|-----|-----|
Not at all   Very much so

Are you a worrier?

|-----|-----|-----|-----|-----|-----|-----|-----|-----|
Not at all   Very much so

If your crosses are, by and large, towards the right end of the line, then you believe that your basic nature makes you prone to stress.

Area 2 Your job

How stressful is your job?

|-----|-----|-----|-----|-----|-----|-----|-----|-----|
Not at all stressful   Very stressful

If the job is stressful, go through these questions to see if you can find the source of the stress. Ask yourself 'Why?' each time:
Workload?

|-----|-----|-----|-----|-----|-----|-----|-----|-----|
Not a problem   Major problem

Nature of the job (e.g. dirty, boring)?

|-----|-----|-----|-----|-----|-----|-----|-----|-----|
Not a problem   Major problem

Are you poorly trained?

|-----|-----|-----|-----|-----|-----|-----|-----|-----|
Not a problem   Major problem

Managers?

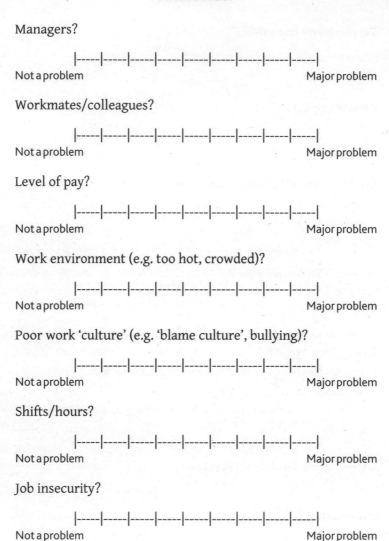

|-----|-----|-----|-----|-----|-----|-----|-----|-----|
Not a problem   Major problem

Workmates/colleagues?

|-----|-----|-----|-----|-----|-----|-----|-----|-----|
Not a problem   Major problem

Level of pay?

|-----|-----|-----|-----|-----|-----|-----|-----|-----|
Not a problem   Major problem

Work environment (e.g. too hot, crowded)?

|-----|-----|-----|-----|-----|-----|-----|-----|-----|
Not a problem   Major problem

Poor work 'culture' (e.g. 'blame culture', bullying)?

|-----|-----|-----|-----|-----|-----|-----|-----|-----|
Not a problem   Major problem

Shifts/hours?

|-----|-----|-----|-----|-----|-----|-----|-----|-----|
Not a problem   Major problem

Job insecurity?

|-----|-----|-----|-----|-----|-----|-----|-----|-----|
Not a problem   Major problem

Travel to and from work?

|-----|-----|-----|-----|-----|-----|-----|-----|-----|
Not a problem   Major problem

Lack of respect?

|-----|-----|-----|-----|-----|-----|-----|-----|-----|
Not a problem   Major problem

Are there any other issues with the job?

Look at your answers. Can you see any way to tackle the sources of stress you have identified? Or, if they can't be changed, can you see a better way of coping with them? Write down any thoughts you may have.

Area 3 Your health

How is your health?

|-----|-----|-----|-----|-----|-----|-----|-----|-----|
Not a problem   Major problem

Why is this?

How much does your health affect your stress?

|-----|-----|-----|-----|-----|-----|-----|-----|-----|
Not at all   A great deal

Why is this?

How much does your stress affect your health?

|-----|-----|-----|-----|-----|-----|-----|-----|-----|
Not at all   A great deal

Why is this?

Is there anything you can do to improve your health? Does anyone else close to you have health problems? Do you help take care of them? How well do you cope with this?

Area 4 Your relationships

Are you unhappy with your home life?

|-----|-----|-----|-----|-----|-----|-----|-----|-----|
Not at all   Very much so

Why?

Are you unhappy with your main relationship(s)?

|-----|-----|-----|-----|-----|-----|-----|-----|-----|
Not at all   Very much so

Why?

Do you feel you lack support around you (e.g. to help with children)?

|-----|-----|-----|-----|-----|-----|-----|-----|-----|
Not at all   Very much so

Why?

Do you have problems trusting those close to you?

|-----|-----|-----|-----|-----|-----|-----|-----|-----|
Not at all   Very much so

Why?

Do those close to you have problems trusting you?

|-----|-----|-----|-----|-----|-----|-----|-----|-----|
Not at all   Very much so

Why?

Do you feel under threat from anyone?

|-----|-----|-----|-----|-----|-----|-----|-----|-----|
Not at all   Very much so

Why?

Does anyone feel under threat from you?

|-----|-----|-----|-----|-----|-----|-----|-----|-----|
Not at all   Very much so

Why?

Do you feel there are people close to you who add to your stress?

|-----|-----|-----|-----|-----|-----|-----|-----|-----|
Not at all   Very much so

Why?

Do you feel there are people close to you who are also under stress?

|-----|-----|-----|-----|-----|-----|-----|-----|-----|
Not at all   Very much so

Why?

Are you unhappy with your friends/social life?

|-----|-----|-----|-----|-----|-----|-----|-----|-----|
Not at all   Very much so

Why?

Are your children causing you problems?

|-----|-----|-----|-----|-----|-----|-----|-----|-----|
Not at all   Very much so

Why?

Do you feel lonely?

|-----|-----|-----|-----|-----|-----|-----|-----|-----|
Not at all   Very much so

Why?

Do you feel there is no one there for you when you need someone?

|-----|-----|-----|-----|-----|-----|-----|-----|-----|

Not at all   Very much so

Why?

Area 5 Your money

Can you see a way to tackle any of these problems?

Is lack of money a problem for you?

|-----|-----|-----|-----|-----|-----|-----|-----|-----|
Not at all   Very much so

Do you have problems with debt?

|-----|-----|-----|-----|-----|-----|-----|-----|-----|
Not at all   Very much so

Are you living beyond your means?

|-----|-----|-----|-----|-----|-----|-----|-----|-----|
Not at all   Very much so

Are your money problems due to someone else's spending?

|-----|-----|-----|-----|-----|-----|-----|-----|-----|
Not at all   Very much so

How does this affect your day-to-day life?

Can you see any way to work on these problems?

Area 6 Your home/neighbourhood

Do you have problems with your neighbours?

|-----|-----|-----|-----|-----|-----|-----|-----|-----|
Not at all   Very much so

Why?

Does your neighbourhood make you stressed?

|-----|-----|-----|-----|-----|-----|-----|-----|-----|
Not at all   Very much so

Why?

Do your living conditions add to your stress (e.g. not enough space, house needs repairs, mortgage/rent too high)?

|-----|-----|-----|-----|-----|-----|-----|-----|-----|
Not at all   Very much so

Can you see any way to deal with the issues?

Area 7 Your behaviour

Is your behaviour giving cause for concern to others?

|-----|-----|-----|-----|-----|-----|-----|-----|-----|
Not at all   Very much so

Why?

Are you bored with your life?

|-----|-----|-----|-----|-----|-----|-----|-----|-----|
Not at all   Very much so

Why?

Do you have problems with drinking, drugs, gambling, smoking, eating? (specify which)

|-----|-----|-----|-----|-----|-----|-----|-----|-----|
Not at all   Very much so

How does this affect your day-to-day life? Can you see any way to deal with these issues?

Area 8 Your strengths

Note that in this area the more to the *right* you place your cross, the *greater* your strengths are.

Would those who know you best say you were a good person?

|-----|-----|-----|-----|-----|-----|-----|-----|-----|
Not at all   Very much so

Are you an honest person?

|-----|-----|-----|-----|-----|-----|-----|-----|-----|
Not at all   Very much so

On the whole, do you live up to the standards you set yourself?

|-----|-----|-----|-----|-----|-----|-----|-----|-----|
Not at all   Very much so

Are you a good family member?

|-----|-----|-----|-----|-----|-----|-----|-----|-----|
Not at all   Very much so

Are you a kind person?

|-----|-----|-----|-----|-----|-----|-----|-----|-----|
Not at all   Very much so

Are you a good friend?

|-----|-----|-----|-----|-----|-----|-----|-----|-----|
Not at all   Very much so

Are you someone who respects other people?

|-----|-----|-----|-----|-----|-----|-----|-----|-----|
Not at all   Very much so

If need be, can you see a way to improve upon your strengths?

Stage 4 Measure your stress and well-being

The GAD-7 scale measures anxiety. The PHQ-9 measures depression. The WEMWBS measures well-being. The higher the score on the first two, the greater the problem. The lower the score on the third, the poorer your well-being. For each of them, circle the number that best describes how you feel and add up your score. You can see how to score beneath each scale. Keep coming back to these scales as you progress though the book to check your progress.

Generalised Anxiety Disorder (GAD-7)*

Over the last two weeks, how often have you been bothered by the following problems?

	Not at all	Several days	More than half the days	Nearly every day
Feeling nervous, anxious or on edge	0	1	2	3
Not being able to stop or control worrying	0	1	2	3
Worrying too much about different things	0	1	2	3
Trouble relaxing	0	1	2	3
Being so restless that it is hard to sit still	0	1	2	3
Becoming easily annoyed or irritable	0	1	2	3

* Developed by Drs Robert L. Spitzer, Janet B. W. Williams, Kurt Kroenke and colleagues, with an educational grant from Pfizer Inc. No permission required to reproduce, translate, display or distribute.

Feeling afraid as if something awful might happen	0	1	2	3

0–4	No anxiety
5–9	Mild anxiety
10–14	Moderate anxiety
15–21	Severe anxiety

Patient Health Questionnaire (PHQ-9)*

Over the last two weeks, how often have you been bothered by any of the following problems?

	Not at all	Several days	More than half the days	Nearly every day
Little interest or pleasure in doing things	0	1	2	3
Feeling down, depressed, or hopeless	0	1	2	3
Trouble falling or staying asleep, or sleeping too much	0	1	2	3

* PHQ-9 Copyright © Pfizer. Reprinted with permission, courtesy of Pfizer Limited.

Feeling tired or having little energy	0	1	2	3
Poor appetite or overeating	0	1	2	3
Feeling bad about yourself, or that you are a failure or have let yourself or your family down	0	1	2	3
Trouble concentrating on things, such as reading the newspaper or watching television	0	1	2	3
Moving or speaking so slowly that other people could have noticed. Or the opposite: being so fidgety or restless that you have been moving around a lot more than usual	0	1	2	3
Thoughts that you would be better off dead, or of hurting yourself in some way.	0	1	2	3

0–4	No depression
5–9	Mild depression
10–14	Moderate depression
15–19	Moderately severe depression
20–27	Severe depression

Bear in mind that scores can vary day by day. However, if you scored highly on the final question or if you fear making an attempt on your life, tell someone how you feel and ask that person to stay with you if possible while you seek professional assistance. Your GP will help; outside surgery hours go straight to your nearest A&E department.

Warwick-Edinburgh Mental Well-Being Scale (WEMWBS)

The Warwick-Edinburgh Mental Well-being Scale is a widely used measure of well-being. In the scoring section, we use the terms 'languishing' (poor well-being) and 'flourishing' (good well-being). We will look at these in detail in Chapter 10.

Below are some statements about feelings and thoughts. Please tick the box that best describes your experience of each over the last two weeks.

	None of the time	Rarely	Some of the time	Often	All of the time
I've been feeling optimistic about the future	1	2	3	4	5
I've been feeling useful	1	2	3	4	5
I've been feeling relaxed	1	2	3	4	5

I've been feeling interested in other people	1	2	3	4	5
I've had energy to spare	1	2	3	4	5
I've been dealing with problems well	1	2	3	4	5
I've been thinking clearly	1	2	3	4	5
I've been feeling good about myself	1	2	3	4	5
I've been feeling close to other people	1	2	3	4	5
I've been feeling confident	1	2	3	4	5
I've been able to make up my own mind about things	1	2	3	4	5
I've been feeling loved	1	2	3	4	5
I've been interested in new things	1	2	3	4	5
I've been feeling cheerful	1	2	3	4	5

Add up your score. Your total score will be between 14 and 70.

Languishing

14–32 points Your well-being score is very low.

33–40 points Your well-being score is below average.

> A score of 40 or below means you are leaning more towards languishing. So work hard at well-being and the other skills you are learning as you work through this book. Take the test in a month or so and see if you are moving in the right direction.

Middling

41–59 points Your well-being score is average.

> A score of 41 to 59 puts you into the middling group. That's fine, but it's still worthwhile to boost this further and move into the flourishing camp.

Flourishing

60–70 points Your well-being score is above average.

Remember, none of this is set in stone – the more you practise your stress control skills, the more your well-being will improve.

Stage 5 Draw your vicious circle

In Chapter 2 we looked at the vicious circle of stress. Using the answers you have given so far, can you now think what your own circle looks like? As you do this, think about what you could do to weaken the circle and start to create your own positive circle.

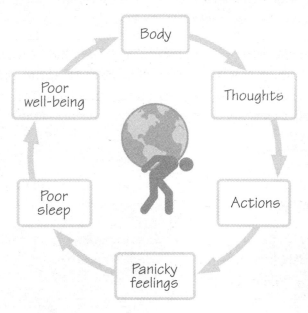

So, starting with your body, write down how it is affected by stress and then ask yourself if you can think of any way to tackle this. Do the same for thoughts and so on till you have completed the circle.

Come back to this page from time to time and, if you need to, amend your answers as you learn more about how stress affects you.

Stage 6 Set your goals

Now that you have worked out how stress affects you and have drawn your own vicious circle, you can set your goals. These should be *clear* and *realistic*.

Good goals, like the ones below, are those where you can clearly measure if you have achieved them. Bad goals don't let you do this.

Bad goals	Good goals
Try to relax more	Keep 30 minutes each night for me to relax
Spend more time with the kids	Have our meals at the table with the family and ask them about their day
Try not to drink as much	Cut alcohol down to two nights each week; no more than four pints each night
Try to get out more	Join the yoga class in the Centre
Try to be a nicer person	Sit down with my partner to try to sort out the problems in the marriage

Now that you know your enemy, see if you can work out some clear goals (write them down) that you can keep in the forefront of your mind as you go on to learn some skills to control your stress. The SMART goals in Chapter 11 will help you to plan how to achieve them.

Last words

The aim of this chapter has been to help you 'know your enemy' and to use that information to attack your stress. It starts the ball rolling for you to 'become your own therapist'. As you achieve your goals, keep setting new ones. Make sure you pat yourself on the back when you succeed. If you fail, don't criticize yourself; stand back and see if there is a better way to achieve them. Use the skills you will learn in this book to help you.

Chapter 4 provides some great self-help ideas to enable you to start tackling your stress.

4

First steps

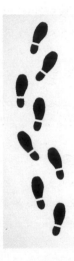

This chapter aims to get you in the best shape before learning the major skills to combat stress. It will help you get rid of the things in your life that may be helping keep stress alive, and then looks at some great self-help ideas with which you can build a sense of control. It is divided into three sections:

- Clearing the decks.
- Finding hidden problems.
- Twenty-five ways to cope.

Clearing the decks

Think of ways to get rid of the things that might be making your stress worse. These may include:

Alcohol/drugs

Many people with a drink problem start down that road by using alcohol to calm their nerves. Having a drink is fine, but if you drink to cope with stress you may start to depend on it. If you can't go to certain places or do certain things unless you have a drink beforehand, you are storing up trouble for yourself.

You may find that you need to use more and more drink as time goes on, or use legal or illegal drugs. Some people use cannabis to relax, for instance, but be aware that overuse of either alcohol or cannabis can lead to feelings of depression, paranoia, anxiety, poor sleep, anger and confusion. Body symptoms such as nausea, sweating, shaking and loss of appetite may be due to drink or drugs rather than stress. So look for better ways to control your stress.

The 'miracle cure'

It does not exist. Stress often takes a long time to build up so it is not going to clear up overnight. Getting on top of stress takes a great deal of hard work on *your* part. So the answer lies within you. This book will put you on the right lines, but at the end of the day only you, through your hard work, can control your stress.

Although they can help you to relax at the time, there is no good evidence to show that alternative therapies such as hypnosis, reiki, acupuncture, aromatherapy or homeopathy are of much use in the long run. By all means use these approaches as they can help in the short term, but don't expect them to sort out your stress. You must learn to control the stress yourself.

Reassurance

This may be nice in the short term, but you can become dependent on it. If you constantly ask people at home or at work for reassurance they may eventually get fed up with you (and may start reassuring you just to shut you up!). This can lead to friction and, hence, more stress. You have to feel strong enough to supply your own answers.

Self-criticism

If people under stress have one great skill, it is this. But tearing strips off yourself doesn't help. If things go wrong, accept them; learn from your mistakes and move on. Pat yourself on the back every time you try to combat your stress. This will help your self-confidence to pick up. Give yourself a break.

Avoidance

Common sense tells us that if doing something makes us more stressed, we should avoid it. **Common sense is wrong.** Avoidance may help in the short term, but in the long run you just build up more trouble for yourself. We all know what to do if we fall off a horse . . . You have to face up to the problems in your life. Facing up to stress will be hard in the short term but, in the long run, will help you to control it (see Chapter 7). The big message is: Face your Fears.

Finding hidden problems

Before you try to control your stress, check in case it is trying to tell you that there is something wrong in your life that you need to sort out. These problems could include:

- Loneliness.
- Gambling.
- Children.
- Parents.
- Friends.
- Work.
- Money.
- Being stubborn.
- Immaturity.
- Being too dependent.

Most people suffering from stress do not have hidden problems, but double check your own situation before moving on. Examples might be:

- Someone close to you has problems that affect you.
- Someone close to you is treating you badly.
- There are problems at work that need to be faced.

- You are living beyond your means.
- There are family issues that need to be dealt with.

There may not be an easy answer to hidden problems, but if you don't face up to them and deal with them they will keep your stress alive.

Twenty-five ways to cope

The following straightforward skills can help while you are learning how to get on top of stress. Read through all these ideas and pick up the skills that best meet your needs.

1 Keep your life as normal as you can You may find that stress invades many areas of your life. Keep a normal routine going even if you don't feel like doing so. If you go to watch football at the weekend, *keep going*; if you visit your mother during the week, *keep going*; if you go to a fitness class twice a week, *keep going*. As work is an important part of our routine, try to keep going to it if you can. Make sure you eat properly prepared meals at the right times. Keeping a structure in your day will help hold back the problems.

2 Deal with problems on the spot Don't bottle up your feelings. They will grow and grow inside you until they finally erupt. This will weaken your sense of control. So if there are problems at work, for example, make sure that you deal with them on the spot.

3 Strong, confiding relationships Stress often makes us harder to live with, and this can weaken relationships. But we know that strong relationships can help fight stress. So if you have a weak relationship and feel it is worth keeping, work hard at fixing it.

4 Slow down Don't do things at 100 miles an hour. Eat, walk and drive more slowly. If you don't get as much done as you would like then it's no big deal. Take your time and remember there are only twenty-four hours in each day. And there is always another day.

5 Divide problems up If you face a huge problem and can see no way to cope with it, see if you can divide it up into smaller 'bite-size' bits. Then tackle them one at a time (see Chapter 7).

6 Look and sound relaxed Other people will pick up on how you are feeling through your body language. So try to look relaxed: don't sit on the edge of your seat, slow down your speech, relax your shoulders, don't fidget. Ask those close to you how you act when you are tense so that you know what changes to make. You will feel better if you know that, on the outside at least, you are looking calm (see number 14 below).

7 Focus on the moment As soon as you feel your stress levels rise, concentrate on what is happening right now. Pick something to focus on: if you are outside, the sound of the birds, an individual leaf; if inside, examine a picture in as much detail as possible. Let other thoughts that come into your mind just drift away.

8 'Must' and 'should' 'I *must* see my mother today'; 'I *should* offer to run the football team this year'. Work out what is reasonable for you to achieve and be happy with your decision: 'If I get through all the things I want to at home, I'll take a run down to my mother's. If not, I'll see her later in the week'; 'I don't get a chance to relax as it is so it's daft to take on more pressure – someone else can take a turn.'

9 Coping with ruts If you feel your life is in a rut just now – same old routine day in, day out – then think about change. Plan your weekends, and do something different: go for a drive, visit friends, go for a long walk. Take up new hobbies. Look for challenges. If you can afford it, plan the odd weekend away, as a change of scenery can help.

10 Mantras Sit alone in a quiet, dark room. Try to clear your mind as much as possible. Think of a word or phrase, such as 'I am calm' or 'Relax' or 'I am in control'. Close your eyes and slowly repeat the word or phrase in your mind over and over again. Do this for ten minutes each day, or when you feel stressed. If unwanted thoughts come into your mind, try not to pay them any attention and just let them drift away (see number 7 above).

11 Build relaxation into your life No matter how busy you are, put aside some time each day just for you. Go out for a walk, phone a friend, tend the garden, read a book, watch TV, listen to music.

12 Past experience If you are in a tricky situation, ask yourself if you have been in a similar jam before. How did you deal with it? If what you did worked, try it again. If it didn't, learn from your mistakes.

13 Don't accept other people's targets Do people expect too much of you? If you feel they do, *confront* this. Have a quiet word and try to sort it out. If you can't agree, say 'No'.

14 Calm breathing Breathe in slowly through your nose for a count of three to four seconds. Hold this for another three to four seconds, then breathe out through your mouth over a count of six to eight seconds. Repeat this three times, every hour.

15 Smoking Some people find that smoking helps them to relax, but it floods the body with nicotine which acts as a stimulant and may increase feelings of stress. Try to stop. Ask your GP for help.

16 Situations beyond your control There are some things in life that you can't change – maybe you can't afford to move house, maybe a loved one is ill, maybe you can't change job. If you accept that you can't do anything to change certain things for the better, this may help reduce the stress that remains.

17 'Worry time' Put aside fifteen minutes in the evening. This is your time to worry about the things that have bothered you in the day. So if you start to worry about something in the morning, stop and tell yourself to store it up for your 'worry time' that night. At the start of your 'worry time' think of what you were going to worry about and then try to do so. You may not even recall what it was. If you do, it may feel not worth worrying about, or hard to bring on.

18 One thing at a time Think of someone at work cradling a phone between his shoulder blade and ear. With one hand he is tapping away at his keyboard, and with the other searching through some papers. At the same time, he is trying to grab a quick snack. He is overloading the system. If you are making a phone call, make only the call and nothing else. The message is: don't keep too many balls in the air at the one time.

19 Other people's shoes Think of a problem you have. Imagine how you would react if a friend came to you with that same problem. What advice would you give them? Would that advice work for you?

20 Do the worst thing first If you have a list of things to do, do the one you least want to do first. Get it out of the way and the remaining tasks will be easier to cope with. If you keep putting it off, it will prey on your mind and may seem a lot worse than it really is. Tie this in with your priority list (see number 23).

21 Don't try to be Superman or Wonder Woman Do you try to do it all? Try to succeed at everything? Want to be the best? Why? Keep in mind that the house or your job will still be there long after you are gone. Stick to your good points and learn to live with your faults. Accept you are not perfect. None of us is.

22 Confide in others If there are people around whom you can trust, let them know how you feel. They may be able to offer good advice that you have not thought about. In any case, getting things off your chest can help. It may also help reduce the feelings of being alone that are so common in stress. Sometimes just having someone listen can help lift your spirits.

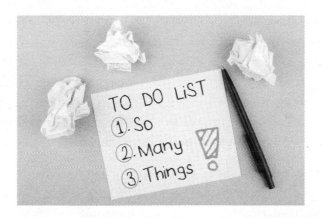

23 Prioritize If you do have a busy life, set up your priorities. Decide what has to be done now and what can wait. Put these tasks in order of priority. 'Number 1 has to be done first thing, number 2 by 12 o'clock . . . number 10 has to be done by the end of the month.' Keep revising your list.

24 Exercise Thirty minutes of exercise, five days a week, can help a lot. *Moderate* exercise is as good as *intense*. 'Moderate' is when you increase your heart rate but can still talk without puffing. A brisk walk is perfect. Chapter 5 will tell you more.

25 One goal a day Try this if you feel you don't have a good structure to the day or if you don't get round to doing things. Each night, work out a goal for the next day: something you are *not* doing but *should* be doing. For example:

- Go to the gym.
- Cut the grass.
- Clean the living room.

- Meet a friend.
- Open and check a bank statement.

In other words, the usual things you would do if you felt on top of things.

Try to make your goals precise – 'cut the grass' *not* 'work in the garden'. This helps you know whether you have achieved what you set out to achieve. If the grass is cut or the gym visited, then you have achieved your goal and a pat on the back is in order.

The aim is for you to go to bed each night being able to say to yourself that you have taken at least one step forward. This will build you up for your next goal.

Last words

The aim of Chapter 4 is to help you take your first steps in the fightback against stress. From now on, you will be learning more powerful skills to fight stress. Chapter 5 teaches you the first major skill – controlling your body. In the meantime, keep fighting the stress using these new skills.

5

Controlling your body

Stress affects your body. And the way your body reacts affects stress. This helps keep stress alive. So controlling your body helps you to control your stress. In this chapter you will learn the skills that will help you do this.

Part 1 Information

Most people with stress go to their GP initially to ask for help with some physical symptom or other. This is no surprise as the body reacts to stress in a vast number of ways. You may find that you are more prone to some signs while never getting others. You might see your stress signs change over time.

They are usually unpleasant and you may become afraid of them. We call this 'a fear of fear': you start to worry about them, and may avoid doing things in an attempt to stop them. So if you fear your heart racing, you might not run for a bus as you know this will push up your heart rate. Of course, the fact you are worried often means that the signs get stronger as a result.

You may find that the signs appear out of the blue when you least expect them. Often they seem to be on a hair trigger and can appear in a split second. To make more sense of the way the body is affected by stress, let's first look at *anxiety*.

Anxiety affects the body in two main ways:

Muscles become tense, resulting in:

- Tight chest.
- Pain at the back of the neck.
- Aches and pains.

Autonomic Nervous System (ANS) speeds up, resulting in:

- Heart racing.
- Feeling breathless.
- Sweating.

Some of the more common signs are listed below. This is by no means complete so don't worry if you have signs that don't appear here. Anxiety is strongly influenced by 'fight/flight' – the system built into all of us to protect us from danger – filling us with energy so that we can either fight the danger or run away. Once stress gets a grip, fight/flight can spark off many times each day. Think of a car alarm that is so sensitive that it gets set off not just when someone breaks a window but when someone brushes against the door – fight/flight in stress is much the same.

Common body signs of anxiety		
Palpitations	Rapid heart rate	Loss of appetite
Missed heart beats	Dizziness	Craving for food
Faintness	Headaches	Flushing/chills
Numbness	Chest pain/tightness	Nausea
Shortness of breath	Stomach pains	Blurred vision
Choking sensation	Muscle aches/pains	Voice tremor
'Butterflies'	Tiredness	'Freezing'
Shakiness	Sweating	Pins and needles
Sleeping problems	Problems swallowing	Feeling unreal
'Jelly legs'	Trembling	Dry mouth
Bladder weakness	Diarrhoea	Clammy hands

Now let's look at common signs of *depression*.

Many physical signs of depression are the same as those of anxiety. But extremes of reaction are more common, e.g. with appetite. You might not want to eat. You might want to eat a lot more (eating for comfort?). This may lead to weight loss or weight gain. Sleep is the same – sometimes you might not be able to get (back) to sleep, or you might want to sleep far too much.

Depression tends to make us feel physical pain – joint or back pains, or chest pains for example – more acutely (see your GP if you have any worries about this).

People with depression often tell me that they never feel well or 100 per cent. You may feel that your body, like your mind, has lost its sharpness. You may feel constantly tired, or exhausted even after mild exertion. You may feel that you have to drag yourself through the day. You don't feel tired because of what you have done; you may feel tired at the thought of what you have to do.

Common body signs of depression		
Eating a lot less	Weight gain	Never feeling 100 per cent
Eating a lot more	Weight loss	Sluggish
Back pains	Joint pains	Nausea
Worsening chronic pain	Menstrual cycle change	Stomach pains
Chest pains	Moving/speaking more slowly	Diarrhoea
Sexual problems	Loss of libido	Migraine
Headaches	Lack of energy	Sleeping a lot more than usual
Aches and pains	Easily tired	Can't get to sleep
Constipation	Feeling exhausted all the time	Waking up during the night
Agitation	Body feels numb	Waking early in the morning

In Chapter 2 we talked about vicious circles. Let's look at how these can build up.

At this early stage, our vicious circle is still being fed, and so remains powerful. But as we learn controlling body skills, we make the first impact on it (and see how the body no longer feeds the circle).

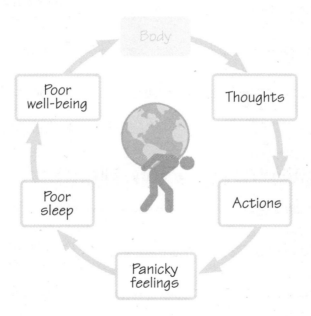

And as we learn skills to control our body, the positive circle, though still very weak, starts to build:

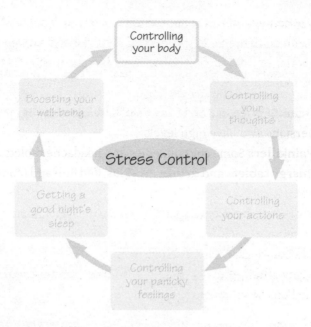

Part 2 Controlling your body skills

There are five skills to be learned in controlling your body:

- Limit caffeine.
- Exercise.
- Breathing retraining.
- Progressive muscular relaxation.
- Healthy eating.

Skill 1 Limit caffeine

Caffeine can help make you feel alert. It can help you concentrate. It can improve your reaction time. It can help keep you going when you need to. But the effects of too much caffeine can be much the same as those of anxiety. It is a stimulant that affects the brain and central nervous system (CNS). Caffeine can be found in:

- **Drinks** Coffee, tea and fizzy drinks like Coke or Pepsi. Diet versions also have high levels.
- **Painkillers** Some cold remedies and headache tablets.
- **Energy tablets and drinks** Pro-Plus, Red Bull and Monster, etc.
- **Workout supplements** May contain large amounts of caffeine.
- **Chocolate** Especially dark varieties.
- Many other products contain caffeine so read the information on the packaging carefully.

The effects of too much caffeine include feeling nervous, irritable, restless, agitated, shaky, having headaches, muscle twitches, flushed face, upset stomach, increased heart rate, speeded up breathing and passing water more frequently than usual.

Taking 150mg of caffeine before you go to bed will make it harder to get to sleep and will affect the quality of your sleep (see the chart below which details how much caffeine is contained in a range of products).

How much is too much?

Some people can take vast amounts of caffeine and seem none the worse for it. A rough rule of thumb is that more than 600mg a day may cause problems, but people who are anxious and prone to panic may react to *much* smaller amounts. So it is worthwhile to look at how much caffeine you take each day. The list below will help you work this out (see www.caffeinein-former.com for more details). If you think caffeine does play a part in your stress, you should reduce your daily intake as much as you can.

Hot drinks	Per mug (in milligrams)
Starbucks Venti (large) latte	150
Starbucks brewed coffee	445
Instant coffee	100
Decaf coffee	6
Tea	85–110

Fizzy drinks	Per can
Coke	36
Diet Coke	46
Pepsi	38
Diet Pepsi	43
Dr Pepper	41

Chocolate	
Milk	22mg per 100g
Plain	72mg per 100g

Tablets	
Panadol Extra	65
Anadin Extra	45

Energy	
Pro-Plus energy tablet	50
Red Bull energy drink (250ml)	80
Monster energy drink (473ml)	160

If you feel you are taking too much caffeine, it is important to reduce it slowly. Your body can get so used to caffeine that if you just cut it out you can suffer withdrawal effects that can last for up to one week:

- Throbbing headache.
- Drowsiness/tiredness.
- Anxiety
- Depression.
- Nausea.

If you want to reduce your caffeine, you should:

- Wean yourself off it slowly. This will stop withdrawal effects.
- Slowly switch to *decaf* tea and coffee.
- Slowly switch from fizzy drinks to caffeine-free drinks or pure fruit juice.
- Avoid energy drinks and tablets.
- Take as few painkillers as you can (ask your GP for advice) or switch to lower caffeine brands.

Skill 2 Exercise

We all know that exercise is good for your health. Benefits include weight control, reducing blood pressure, helping to keep bones, muscles and joints healthy, improving body shape, possibly staving off some forms of dementia and reducing the risk of heart disease, diabetes and some cancers.

So exercise makes sense if you want to stay fit. And we now know that exercise can also help fight stress (this fits with the 'healthy body, healthy mind' model in Chapter 1). You may have found that you feel better after exercise. This is good, but to get long-lasting benefit you need to do regular exercise. It needn't cost a lot: a brisk walk, running or swimming are all easily accessible (and cheaper than going to the gym or joining a golf club).

Make sure you choose something you like. You could do a range of things to give you a bit of variety. Bear in mind that if you do go to the gym it gets you out of the house and puts you in contact with other people. This can help in itself.

Why does exercise help stress?
We know that it does, but we are not sure how it works. There are a few theories:

- It boosts serotonin in the brain and this reduces distress.
- It boosts endorphins ('feel-good' hormones) and these boost our sense of well-being.
- It helps boost self-esteem by giving us new goals and a renewed sense of purpose.

How much time do I need to spend? You should try to do at least thirty minutes most days of the week.

Does this have to be at the one time? No. You can break it up. You could spread it across the day by doing fifteen minutes in the morning and fifteen minutes later on. If you don't sleep well, try to avoid exercising in the three hours before going to bed as it may make it harder to get to sleep.

How hard must the exercise be? The guidelines say that moderate exercise is as good for you as more intense exercise.

What does that mean? It involves two things:

- You should be aware of your heart rate rising . . .
- . . . but you should not be so out of breath that you could not talk easily (or sing a song).

A brisk walk is termed as moderate, and as good as any other form of exercise.

Do I need to be fit to start this? No. But you should check with your GP if you are unsure. It is best to build up slowly, so you might think of starting with daily short walks.

Do you have to be young to start this? No. All of us can be helped by this. If your GP has no concerns and you start at the right level, age is of no concern.

One other thing To go along with the exercise, please make sure you move every twenty minutes during the day. So if you are sitting in front of the TV, stand up and stretch when the adverts are on.

Getting started is the hardest bit. Once you get into your stride you should find yourself looking forward to exercise. But it is getting started that is often the big challenge. So ask yourself the following:

- How could exercise help me?
- What are the main things stopping me, and how can I overcome them?

Why not start with fifteen-minute walks twice a day? Make sure your heart rate is up and you are on your way.

Skill 3 Belly breathing

Belly breathing is a good way of relaxing your body, and is especially good for controlling feelings of panic. Practise several times a day. You might want to listen to a free audio guide to the belly breathing technique on my website – www. stresscontrolaudio.com.

The main benefit of this technique is that you learn how to breathe from the diaphragm:

- Place one hand on your chest and the other over your belly button.
- As you breathe in, the hand on your stomach should be pushed out while the hand on your chest should not move.
- As you breathe out, your stomach should pull in. Your chest should not move.

To help, breathe in through your nose, purse your lips and breathe out slowly through your mouth. If you are a chest breather, you may find this difficult at first. Lie on your back on the floor as it is easier to do in this position.

Put these two exercises together and do them twice a day. Once you get good at it you can practise when you are at work, sitting on the bus, watching TV, and so on – no matter where you are. No one will notice what you are doing.

This technique is summarized below.

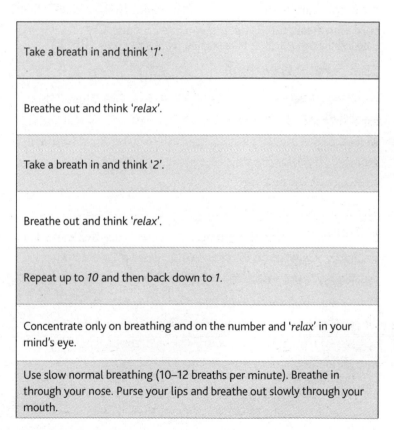

Take a breath in and think '*1*'.

Breathe out and think '*relax*'.

Take a breath in and think '*2*'.

Breathe out and think '*relax*'.

Repeat up to *10* and then back down to *1*.

Concentrate only on breathing and on the number and '*relax*' in your mind's eye.

Use slow normal breathing (10–12 breaths per minute). Breathe in through your nose. Purse your lips and breathe out slowly through your mouth.

Use the diaphragm – as you breathe in, your stomach should push out while your chest should not move.

As you breathe out, your stomach should pull in. Your chest should not move when you breathe out.

Practise twice a day in different places.

Skill 4 Progressive Muscular Relaxation (PMR)

Earlier in this chapter we saw that anxiety affects the body in two ways: it tenses muscles and speeds up the ANS. PMR is a good skill to have because:

- It teaches you to relax the muscles.
- By controlling your breathing it slows down the autonomic nervous system.

These two skills will teach you how to control your body. Audio clips of deep and quick relaxation exercises are available, free of charge and spoken by the author, at www.stresscontrolaudio.com. Written instructions can be found in Appendix 1.

PMR divides into three parts:

- Deep relaxation.
- Quick relaxation.
- Prevention.

Part 1 Deep relaxation

Deep relaxation is the form most favoured by experts in stress control. One word of warning: if you have any problems such as a back injury and are concerned that PMR might make it worse, ask your GP for advice.

What is it? PMR teaches you how to relax your body and mind. You first become aware of the way stress affects your body (*'I didn't realize that my shoulders were up at my ears all day'*), and then you use the track to get rid of it. Once you get good at it, you will be able to detect stress creeping into your body at a much earlier stage. So you will be able to nip it in the bud.

Like all skills it takes a bit of time to pick up PMR; maybe a few weeks to even start feeling relaxed. Bear in mind you are learning something you have lost or never had in the first place. So be patient.

Where should you use the technique? Do it in a room where you can get some peace and quiet and where you can be warm and comfy. Try different rooms to see which is best for you. *Don't* play the audio track while driving your car, for obvious reasons.

Should you sit or lie down? Suit yourself. The best places may be the bed or the sofa, but you may prefer the floor. If you have a comfy chair (recliners are very good), you could use this.

When should you use this technique? Every day. Many people under stress find it hard to find time for PMR, but you must work at this. Decide what time of day suits you best and then stick to it.

What will happen when I play the audio clip? If you use the clip on my website, you will hear my voice. You will tense and relax various muscles. The idea is that you become aware of the difference between tension and relaxation in your muscles. I will then lead you to slow your breathing to a steady pace.

Towards the end of the track, you will move on to ways to relax your mind. After I stop talking, you could just stay where you are to enjoy the relaxed feeling. You count back from four to one to end.

Please note that this is not a hypnotic track so don't worry about going into a trance. You will be in complete control.

Ten tips to help you relax

1 Get as comfy as you can before you start. Take off your shoes and wear loose clothes.

2 Make sure the room is warm. Switch your phone off.

3 Make sure no one in the house comes into the room while you play the track. If they want to join in from the start, that's fine.

4 At first you should do this exercise when you are feeling fairly calm. Just as it is much easier to swim in a calm sea, you will find relaxation easier when you feel calmer. You will be able to concentrate better. This will enable you to pick up the skill more quickly.

5 When you start the exercise you may be thinking of all the other things you should be doing instead. This is a common problem in stress. Do not become distracted. You must set aside time to relax.

6 As with learning any skill, practice makes perfect. So repeat the exercise each day. Try to do it at the same time.

7 Don't worry about how well or badly you are doing. Most people find that their concentration wanders during the first few weeks. This is normal; as you get used to the exercise, it will improve. Let relaxation come naturally; don't try to rush it. When the feeling comes, enjoy it.

8 Use your breathing retraining skills to boost the relaxation. Practise slowing down to about ten to twelve breaths per minute at various times of the day (use the second hand on your watch). This will help you keep your body calm right through the day.

9 PMR can leave you feeling nicely drowsy. Some people fall asleep. If you are one of these don't worry, but bear in mind that you are learning a skill and will get more out of it if you can stay awake. If you need to be alert after the exercise, e.g. driving, make sure that you feel fully on the ball before setting off.

10 You may find that when you tense your muscles, you hold your breath. Don't worry; most people do this at the start. Try to keep the muscle tensing and breathing control separate.

If you want to check on whether you are making progress, keep a diary. Fill it in each time you use the relaxation. Rate your stress level before and after using a 1–10 scale, where '10' means your stress could not be worse. Keep hold of these ratings to see if things improve the more often you use the relaxation.

Keep practising the exercise until you can relax well. You can then switch to the quick relaxation exercise.

Part 2 Quick relaxation

This lets you fine-tune your new skills. The idea is the same as before, except that now you can learn to relax more quickly. It is simply a quick version of what you have just learned. The same rules apply – do the exercise at the same time each day. As before, don't expect to pick it up at once. Don't be put off when it doesn't work first time. See the Appendix for a detailed description of the technique.

If you want to do both exercises each day, then go ahead: you can't get enough relaxation. But the whole aim of PMR is, of course, to teach you a way to control your stress. You should aim to phase out these exercises (you may get bored with them in any case). So your final job is prevention.

Part 3 Prevention

Once you have learned how to relax, try to do it without using the exercises or audio clips, i.e. slot the skill into your brain and retrieve it whenever you need it. With the aid of your newfound skill you can go into stressful situations armed with a new weapon. You now have a way of staying in control. As you will be more alert to stress building up, you can nip it in the bud before it gets the chance to get a grip on you.

You do not have to run through all the parts of the exercises. Stick to the bits you find best for you. This could be breathing control, relaxing your shoulders, and so on. If you are in company do the exercises that no one will notice.

In summary, you should:

Start with deep relaxation/keep a diary.
Practise the exercise every day until you learn to relax.
Move to quick relaxation.
Practise the exercise every day until you can relax quickly.
Move to doing it on your own.
The aim is to nip stress in the bud by relaxing at the very first sign of it building up in your body.

Skill 5 Healthy eating

We've looked at the importance of exercise, keeping alcohol or drug use low and cutting down on caffeine. So to round off achieving a healthy body/healthy mind we will look at the benefits of a healthy diet*.

Eating well can help prevent serious illnesses like heart disease, diabetes or many cancers, high blood pressure and so on. While a poor diet doesn't in itself cause stress, it can add to it. So as part of the range of new skills you have already picked up by reading this book, you should also think about what you eat.

The three main constituents of food are:

Fats

Fats store energy; they keep us warm. They may play a role in keeping stress levels down.

Go for a diet rich in:

- **Unsaturated fats** Seeds, nuts, avocados, vegetable oils like olive and sunflower.
- **Omega-3 fatty acids** Flaxseed, walnuts and oily fish (e.g. mackerel, salmon and trout).

Try to cut back on:

- **Saturated fats** Full-fat milk, butter, cream, cheese, ice-cream, pies.

---

* I will offer general advice but, of course, each person has their own needs. Some illnesses and conditions, e.g., if pregnant or breastfeeding, will require specific recommendations so always have a word with your doctor or dietician for specific advice.

- **Products which often contain trans-fats** Margarine and spreads, cake mixes, biscuits, chips, instant soups and sauces.

Carbohydrates

Carbohydrates act as fuel for the body, especially the brain and muscles.

Try to avoid:

- **Simple carbs** Table sugar, brown sugar, honey, fruit drinks, fizzy drinks, some sports drinks, sweets, jam. These can give you a quick energy boost but it is short-lived.

Go for a diet rich in:

- **Complex carbs** Green veg, whole grains, e.g. oatmeal, pasta, brown or basmati rice, wholegrain bread, potatoes, sweet potatoes, corn, couscous, beans, lentils, peas. These 'good-carb' foods tend to be high in fibre and provide the body with long-term energy.

Proteins

Proteins act as the building blocks of the body and are involved in almost every function of our bodies.

Go for a diet rich in:

- Whole grains, lentils, peas, beans, fish, lean meat, chicken, eggs, nuts, skimmed or semi-skimmed milk.

Supplements

The current advice is that, unless you have a very poor diet, or if your doctor has advised it, you are unlikely to benefit from taking supplements. A balanced diet should provide everything your body needs. Although a wide range of supplements is suggested for stress, the evidence for most is poor or non-existent. Taking too many supplements can be harmful.

A balanced diet

The UK Food Standards Agency suggests the healthiest diet is one where you get the balance right. It recommends:

- Base your diet on starchy foods (potatoes, bread, cereals, couscous, brown rice and pasta).
- Moderate amounts of milk.
- Fish twice a week (at least one should be oily fish such as mackerel or salmon).
- Five portions of fruit and veg each day (fresh, frozen, canned or dried fruit).
- Cut down on salt, saturated fat and sugar.
- Avoid processed food as much as possible.
- Men should drink about 2 litres (3.5 pints) of fluids a day. Women should try for 1.6 litres (just under 3 pints) a day. Drink more on hot days or if exercising more. All fluids count including tea and coffee but water, milk and fruit juices are best.

Last words

The aim of Chapter 5 is to control the body; to start starving the vicious circle and feeding the positive circle. Chapter 6 now adds to the skills you have learned by teaching you to control your thoughts.

6

Controlling your thoughts

Stress affects the way we think. And the way we think affects stress. This helps keep stress alive. So controlling your thoughts helps you to control your stress. This chapter will give you the skills you need to do this.

Part 1 Information

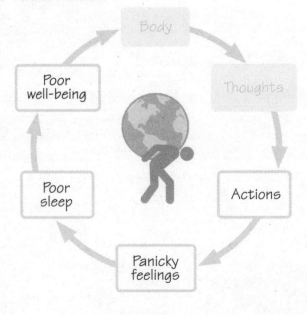

As we learn skills to control our thoughts and combine them with the 'controlling your body' skills, the vicious circle weakens further.

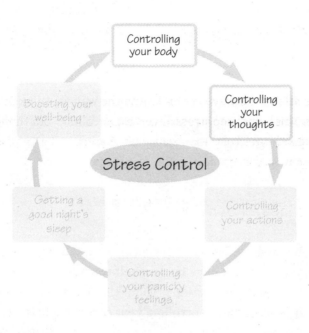

And by combining the 'controlling your body' and 'controlling your thoughts' skills, we can start to starve the vicious circle by slowly strengthening the positive circle.

Stressed thinking

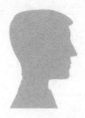

'I just feel so empty inside. I feel so worthless. I want people to like me but there is not much there to like. I just get in the way at work. I'm letting the team down. They must be so fed up with me.'

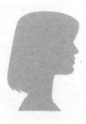

'The second I walk into college each morning, my mind goes into overdrive. What if this happens? What if that happens? Always assuming the worst is going to happen. I know I always look happy, but if only they could see what was going on inside my head all day.'

Imagine thinking like these two people day after day. Think of the impact it would have on your self-confidence, self-esteem, your body and your actions. Thoughts play a crucial role in keeping stress alive. Controlling your thoughts plays a crucial part in getting back in control.

The more common stress thoughts are listed in the chart below.

Common stress thoughts		
Loss of self-confidence	Fear of challenges	Self-criticism
Feeling hopeless	Loss of interest in sex	Mind going blank
Worrying too much	Feeling tense	Sadness
Irritation	Poor concentration	Fear of illness/disease
Loss of interest	Easily confused	Feeling life is a struggle
Afraid to face the day	Feeling worthless	Self-hatred
Feeling that no one understands you	Fear of making a fool of yourself	Too concerned about checking or cleaning
Feeling keyed up or on edge	Feeling cut off from the world	Thoughts about death
Mind going blank	Brooding	Loss of sense of humour
Feeling self-conscious	Loss of interest	Forgetful
Fear of losing control	Feeling guilt keenly	Low self-esteem
Nightmares	Lack of satisfaction	Feeling bad about the world
Fear of being alone	Forgetful	Feel the future is black

Fear of meeting people	Feeling flat	Fear of being criticized
Irritation	Loss of pleasure	Fear of being rejected
Easily startled/on edge	Easily confused/ flustered	Fear of death
Not able to relax	Loss of self-confidence	Easily embarrassed
Self-criticism	Fear of making mistakes	Fear of madness
Fear of the future	Not able to assert yourself	Feeling of impending doom

Stress affects every part of our thinking. When we are stressed we tend to worry about the same things as everyone else: our health, the health of those close to us, our jobs, money and social life. But we worry *much* more and feel unable to stop worrying even when we try to. And we often *worry about worrying* – 'Why am I worrying about this? What's wrong with me?'

'What if' and 'If only'

When we feel down or depressed we often tend to brood on the past (the 'if onlys'), and when we are anxious we often worry about the future (the 'what ifs').

The **if onlys** sometimes involve the loss of something important, e.g.:

- 'If only my mother hadn't died when she did.'
- 'If only I had got that job.'
- 'If only we hadn't moved here.'
- 'If only my partner hadn't left me.'

You might find yourself brooding over these past events for hours.

The **what ifs** are about trying to predict the future, but stress tends to make us *overestimate* the chances of bad things happening and *underestimate* our ability to cope.

- 'What if I can't cope?'
- 'What if I don't know what to say?'
- 'What if I lose my job?'
- 'What if there is something wrong with my heart?'

Common sense voice versus stress voice

When we are stressed it can seem as if there is a non-stop fight going on inside our heads between a loud, abrasive stress voice and a quiet, common sense voice. When we are calm we can listen to our common sense voice, but when we are stressed the loud stress voice drowns it out.

> 'This is awful, I can't cope with this. I'm making a fool of myself here. They all think I'm stupid.'

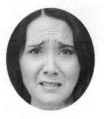

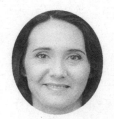

'Get a grip here. I've coped with this in the past. I'm doing OK. Don't get things out of proportion. I can handle this.'

When our stress is high we find it hard to ignore that loud stress voice. And, although we can still hear our common sense voice, it is so quiet and indistinct that we can't really grab hold of it: our stress voice demands to be listened to. Controlling your thoughts is about changing this balance. We will look at how to turn down the volume on this stress voice and learn to listen to our common sense voice until we know, in our heart of hearts, that we can believe it. This will give us a powerful way to control stress.

Vigilance, interpretations, grasshoppers and blinkers

When we feel stressed we usually know we are getting things out of proportion, seeing things as worse than they are or getting uptight about something that we really know isn't going to be as bad as we fear. To deal with this we first of all need to understand what happens when our minds get stressed.

Vigilance

In Chapter 5 we looked at the role of fight/flight – when our bodies and minds are put on alert for detecting and dealing with threats. One of the changes relates to *vigilance*. Let's look at how this works in practice.

Think of a ship sailing through Arctic waters – the ship's radar scans the seas for icebergs (a threat). When the radar detects an iceberg, the captain steers a course into safe waters. The radar rarely sees threats where none exist. We too have a 'radar' that scans for threats. This is very helpful when real threats exist, but once stress gets a grip our radar becomes much too sensitive and detects threats when none exist. If you are under stress, you may well 'see' icebergs everywhere.

This also means that you are blind to the safe waters in between the icebergs and can't see anywhere safe to steer into. So you feel surrounded by problems. This leads you to feeling easily overwhelmed and as if you have little control.

Interpretation

Most of life is not as clear-cut as the example of the iceberg in the path of a ship. That is black and white – icebergs and ships do not mix – whereas our lives are lived in shades of grey. Most things that happen to us have to be *interpreted*:

- What did my manager mean when she said that to me?
- Why is my heart speeding up?
- Why didn't Ian want to come for a coffee with me?

We are much more likely to interpret events as threatening when we are stressed. Maybe there is a better, more reasonable, way to interpret things that happen to us. There is – and to get the ball rolling we need to look at:

Grasshopper thinking

Grasshoppers have one great skill – taking huge physical leaps. When we are stressed, we act like grasshoppers in that we take huge leaps too, but in our thinking. Each leap is bigger than the last, and stress levels can quickly go through the roof:

My pulse is a bit fast.

Oh no, what if there is something wrong with my heart?

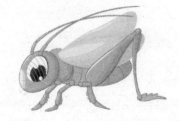

What if I die?

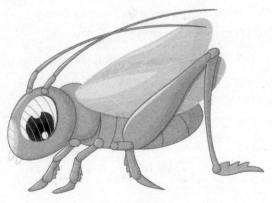

How will my children cope without their mother?

Three increasingly large 'leaps'. Imagine how distressed you could get in a matter of seconds if you have grasshopper thoughts like this? And think how this feeds itself:

- **Because** you are stressed, fight/flight gets triggered.
- **Because** fight/flight is triggered, your heart speeds up and you become more vigilant.
- **Because** you become more vigilant, you focus more on your heart.
- **Because** you focus on your heart, it speeds up more.
- **Because** your heart speeds up, your stress level rises and you become more worried that something serious is wrong.
- **Because** your stress level rises . . . and on and on it goes.

So the way you think affects your body and feeds the vicious circle we saw in Chapter 2. However, as we learn skills to control our thoughts and combine them with controlling your body skills, the vicious circle weakens.

Blinkers

Think of a horse race – the trainer wants the horse to focus only on the track ahead right up to the winning line. So he puts blinkers on the horse so that it doesn't get distracted by the other horses, by the people shouting in the stands, and so on. Now the horse *knows* there are other horses, *knows* there are people in the stands, but isn't really able to pay attention to them because of the blinkers.

This is how stress affects us. This is why understanding the stress voice and the common sense voice is so important.

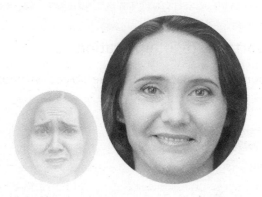

When we are calm, we can listen to our common sense voice and can ignore the stress voice.

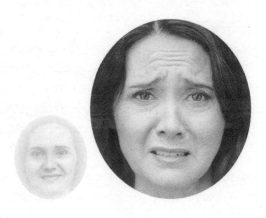

But when we are stressed and the blinkers are on, it is much harder to pay attention to our common sense voice as it is now on the 'wrong side' of the blinkers. It can easily be drowned out by our very loud stress voice which is right in our face. We *know* the common sense is there, but we find it really hard to grab hold of it.

The importance of interpretation

A neighbour walks past you in the street without saying hello. Think of how these two *interpretations* would affect you:

- 'She ignored me on purpose.'
- 'She must be in a hurry; she didn't even see me.'

If you are stressed, you are more likely to interpret what happened as threatening: 'She ignored me on purpose.' If you were calm, you are more likely to interpret the event as non-threatening: 'She must be in a hurry; she didn't even see me.'

That first interpretation sets the ball rolling and feeds your stress. None of us likes to be ignored, so it is understandable that you might be upset. So it is not the way you react to the thought that is wrong, but whether the thought is right in the first place. Did you interpret the event in an accurate way?

Once stress gets a grip, you often accept the interpretation at face value. You don't challenge it because of the blinkers. And if you don't challenge it, it will feed your stress. It would also lead you to search for a reason for her ignoring you. Stress would then kick in and make things even worse.

More thoughts would follow as the grasshopper starts to leap and the level of threat grows. You now have a vicious circle with thoughts feeding stress, stress feeding thoughts and so on. Each thought, because it is not challenged, lets the grasshopper jump to a more stressed thought. This lets the stressed voice get louder and louder. Look at how this works:

Event: Neighbour walks past me

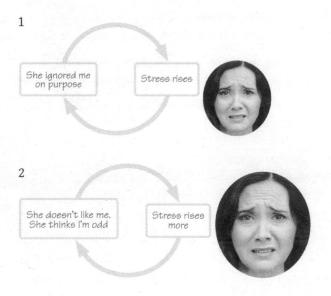

1

She ignored me on purpose → Stress rises

2

She doesn't like me. She thinks I'm odd → Stress rises more

3

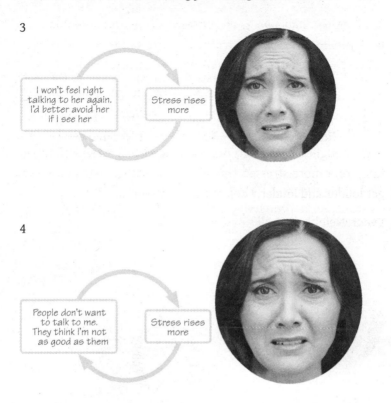

4

You can see how the pattern is set, with thoughts making stress worse and stress making thoughts worse. But note how other things are dragged in. Her *actions* will change – she will avoid talking to the woman. She may avoid going to those shops at times when she thinks the woman might be there. She will avoid talking to others as she feels they will think the same way towards her. Her *body* will react – she will feel uptight leaving her house. And it becomes more general – it now affects everyone, not just the woman who she thinks ignored her.

And all this was set in motion by her interpretation of this one event. How does she know the woman ignored her on purpose? She needs to stand back and challenge the way she views things. Controlling her thoughts would teach her how to do this.

Had she pulled back the blinkers, in what other ways could she have interpreted what happened?

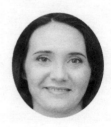 'She must be in a hurry; she didn't even see me.'

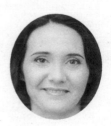 'She did see me. Maybe she is shy and didn't feel up to talking. I can feel like that sometimes.'

'Maybe she is having bad day and doesn't want to talk. I can feel like that.'

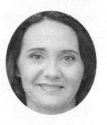

'Maybe she doesn't like me – never mind, you can't be loved by everyone.'

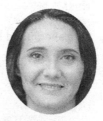

Look at the difference this would make to the vicious circle (and would not trigger stressed actions and body).

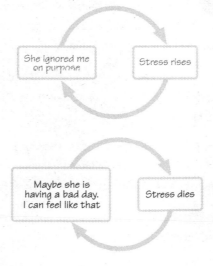

She ignored me on purpose

Stress rises

Maybe she is having a bad day. I can feel like that

Stress dies

In the latter case, the common sense interpretation stops the stress and, as a result, stops the grasshopper from leaping, and so the stress dies.

So you can see that there is usually a range of ways to interpret an event – some good, some bad, most somewhere in between. Controlling your thoughts looks at finding the most *accurate* interpretation so that, in your heart of hearts, you can believe your common sense voice.

How does this help us control stress?

It comes down to turning down the volume of the stress voice and turning up the volume of our common sense voice. The first step in doing this is to pull back the *blinkers* and *build the foundation*.

Once the blinkers are pulled back and we've stopped the *grasshopper thinking*, we stop the stress dead in its tracks by going to the second step and *challenging our thoughts*.

And the good news is that, once you are aware of how these are affecting you, you can learn how to prevent stress in the future by nipping it in the bud. And you do this by learning:

- How to prepare to handle a stressful situation.
- How to cope when you are in that situation.
- How to review how it went to build up your resilience.

So the third and final step is learning to break stress up, which will be covered later in this chapter.

Part 2 Controlling your thoughts skills

Building the foundation

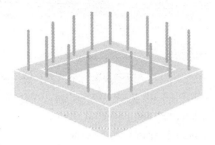

The Big 5 Challenges

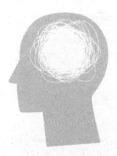

Breaking stress up

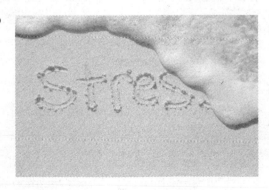

Building the foundation

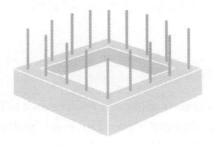

The skills section below teaches you how to challenge your thoughts. Now that may sound like teaching your granny to suck eggs – when we get stressed we do little else but argue with, and feel confused by, our stressed thoughts. But most of the time it fails and we get disheartened. But our challenges collapse because we have not built the foundation properly.

We need a solid foundation upon which we can build our challenges. This lets our common sense voice be heard, allowing us to challenge the stress voice until we can truly believe our common sense voice. Building the foundation is very straightforward, but it is crucial that you put it into place *before* you challenge your thoughts.

It divides into three: **Stand back, pull back the blinkers, wait a minute**. The best way to remember this is to imagine yourself:

Standing back.
Pulling back the blinkers from your face so that you can see the whole picture and let your common sense voice be heard.

Thinking **'wait a minute'** to stop the grasshopper thinking in its tracks, allowing time to move on to the next step, the Big 5 Challenges.

The Big 5 Challenges

Once the foundation is in place, the next step is to learn ways to challenge your thoughts. Once again this is pretty straightforward, but you will need to put in a lot of practice in order to get to grips with it. It grounds the grasshopper by getting your common sense voice back on top. This is achieved by using one of the Big 5 challenges:

1 **What are the chances?** This challenge assumes that the things you worry about are *unlikely* to happen.
2 **What is the worst thing?** This challenge assumes that the things you worry about might well happen but that you may be making too much of them. It looks at keeping a lid on the stress.
3 **The court case** This challenge assumes there is no black-and-white answer here – that it lies in the shades of grey. It works like a court case where the jury has to weigh the evidence and come up with a balanced judgement.
4 **The five-year rule** This challenge assumes that the thing you are worrying about *has* happened or *will* happen. It then asks you to stand back from it and work out how bad it really is.

5 **What is this worth?** This is a great challenge for those everyday stressed thoughts that niggle away at us. It asks us to puts things into perspective.

The challenge you use depends on the stressful thoughts. The more you practise, the easier it will be to pick the right challenge. Look at the following examples of each of the Big 5 Challenges:

What are the chances? (or 'putting your money where your moth is')

This challenge assumes that the things you worry about are *unlikely* to happen. So it asks you how much of your own money would you bet on it happening. Before challenging, it is crucial to build the foundation.

Amy works in a team of twelve people. Once a week, she has to attend a team meeting in a small, claustrophobic room. She is prone to panic and this is one of the worst places for her to go. Her stress voice *screams*:

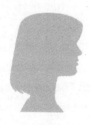

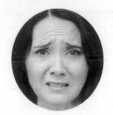

'If I don't get out of here, I'm going to faint.'

Amy needs to challenge her stress before the grasshopper thinking kicks in. So Step 1 is:

Build the foundation: stand back, pull back the blinkers, wait a minute.

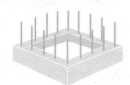

And with the foundation firmly in place, Step 2 is:

Challenge

> 'What are the chances of me fainting? I always think that I am going to faint, yet I never have since I was pregnant. On the few times when I haven't been able to get out, I have felt very faint but then the feeling passed and I was OK. So just stay and brave it out. I'll be fine.'

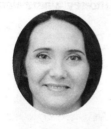

Now that may look a lot simpler than it is. So let's do it again, this time showing every step in more detail.

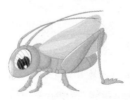

Amy works in a team of twelve people. Once a week, she has to attend a team meeting in a small, claustrophobic room.

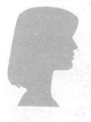

She is prone to panic and this is one of the worst places for her to go. She often tries to find an excuse to get out of going.

She knows she has to try to go to the meeting. Her stress level starts rising the night before at home. She doesn't sleep well and, all morning, gets more and more uptight. She can't concentrate on anything but the upcoming meeting.

Fight/flight is set off on the way to the meeting; her body reacts and she is highly *vigilant*, looking for (and finding) threats, focusing on her faster breathing, faster heart rate and dizziness. By the time she walks into the meeting room, her stress level is already high.

Her first stressed thought is:

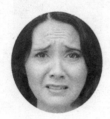

'If I don't get out of here I'm going to faint.'

This is the loud stress voice at full volume. The *blinkers* are firmly on, so while Amy *knows* there are better ways to think about this, she can't access them; her common sense voice seems indistinct and weak as the stress voice drowns it out and overwhelms her.

This is the critical point. If she does not challenge this stressed thought, she will start *grasshopper thinking* with one thought leading quickly to another that is even worse. Things will quickly spiral out of control. She will panic and flee from the meeting, feeding her stress. Her self-esteem and self-confidence will get mauled once again, e.g.:

'If I don't get out of here, I'm going to faint.'

'I'll make a complete fool of myself.'

'My workmates will have had enough of me.
This must embarrass them.'

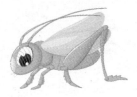

'The boss will find a way to get rid of me.'

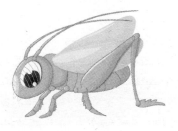

'I'll never get a job again.'

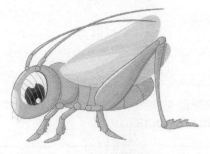

'What's wrong with me, I'm just so useless.'

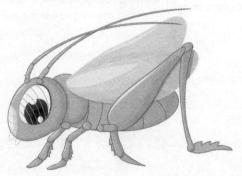

How does Amy pull this back and stay in control? Her first step is to:

Build the foundation:

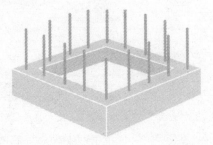

Stand back, pull back the blinkers, wait a minute

Amy imagines herself **standing back, pulling back the blinkers** so that she can see the whole picture. By building the foundation, this gives her the chance to really listen to her common sense voice as it stops the grasshopper thinking in its tracks. This gives her a greater sense of control as she moves to the second step.

Amy then needs to choose the best challenge for this stressed thought. She has five options:

What is the worst thing?	OK, but she never does faint in the meeting so not the best challenge.
The court case	'Weighing the evidence' would work well.
The five-year rule	Nothing really bad is likely to happen so this isn't a good challenge for this particular thought.
What is this worth?	Puts things into perspective. Could work but . . .
What are the chances?	This one is perfect . . .

'What are the chances of me fainting? I always think that I am going to faint, yet I never have since I was pregnant. On the few times when I haven't been able to get out, I have felt very faint but then the feeling passed and I was OK. So just stay calm

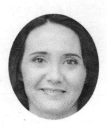

and brave it out. Get my breathing under control. I'll be fine.'

This is Amy's common sense voice talking. Because she has pulled back the blinkers she can hear it clearly and, in her heart of hearts, believes it. By doing this, her stressed voice is now a lot quieter and no longer overwhelms her as it is no longer as believable. She also uses a skill she learned in Chapter 5 – belly breathing. By doing these things, she stopped the grasshopper thinking and so stopped the stress building up. She stays in control and is able to get to, and stay in, the meeting.

She will probably be pretty stressed but it will be at a level she can cope with and so control. As a result, her self-esteem and self-confidence get the chance to start to rebuild. With this victory under her belt the next meeting will be that bit easier as she once again uses the skills she has learned to fight back against the stress. She will stop dreading the meetings as much as she now believes in her own ability to cope. She is becoming her own therapist.

So you can see that controlling stressful thoughts does not happen by chance. You have to firstly understand how stress gets a grip, and then learn the control skills. Then *practise, practise, practise.* It can be useful, at least at first, to use a Thoughts Practice Form (see below).

Let's look at other challenges and, with each, bear in mind all the steps we have shown with Amy.

Big 5 Challenge

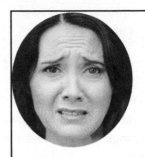

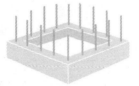

Stand back, pull back the blinkers, wait a minute.

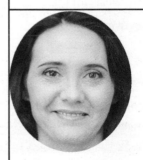

What is the worst thing? (or 'putting a lid on it')

This challenge assumes that the things you worry about might well happen but that you may be making too much of them. So you learn to put a lid on the stress.

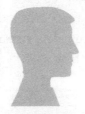 Gerry finds that his concentration is awful due to stress. He has become more self-conscious when meeting clients and this is his stress voice:

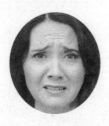 'What if I forget all the details of the product? I'll come across like an idiot.'

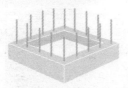 **Build the foundation: stand back, pull back the blinkers, wait a minute.**

Challenge

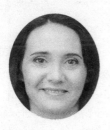 '**What is the worst thing** that can happen? The worst thing is that I'll forget some details. Big deal – I'll look them up on my tablet. I may not come across like the world's greatest salesman but I won't look like the worst. I've forgotten details in the

past and have looked them up and still made the sale. It's no big deal. Keep things in proportion.'

The court case (or 'weighing the evidence')
This challenge assumes there is no black-and-white answer – that it lies in the shades of grey. It works like a court case where the jury has to weigh the evidence and come up with a balanced judgement. It asks 'Am I right to think that . . .?'

Carol has been prone to low self-esteem for some years. She finds it very hard to pat herself on the back but is very good at tearing strips off herself when she thinks something has gone wrong. This is her stress voice (just think of the effect this voice would have on her self-esteem):

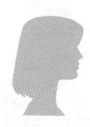

'I'm a failure.'

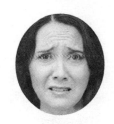

Build the foundation: stand back, pull back the blinkers, wait a minute.

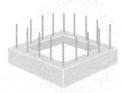

Challenge

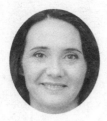

'**Am I right to think that I'm a failure?** I know I shout at the kids a lot but stress makes me do this. I try my best, and a lot of the time I can be OK. I'm holding down my job – just – but I'm still coping. I ask too much of myself – I can't be perfect. I'm far from it but I'm not the worst by a long way. On balance, I'm doing OK.'

The five-year rule (or 'the history game')

This challenge assumes that the thing you are worrying about *has* happened or *will* happen. It then asks you to stand back from it and work out how bad it really is. You ask yourself 'How much will this matter in five years' time?'

Samira gets easily overwhelmed and, when she does, tends to make a lot of mistakes. In this particular situation she did, in truth, make a real mess of things. She felt ashamed and embarrassed. This is her stress voice:

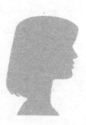

'I really messed things up this morning. I made such a fool of myself. I'm not going back.'

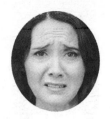

Build the foundation: stand back, pull back the blinkers, wait a minute.

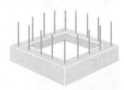

Challenge

'How much will this matter in five years' time? Get things in perspective here. It was awful this morning but it is over and I'm still on my feet. I've learned something and it won't happen again. If that is the worst thing to happen to me for the next five years, then I will be lucky. Stick in there.

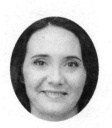

There isn't much chance of it happening again, but if it does I'll know how to handle it better.'

What is this worth? (or 'is life too short?')

This is a great challenge for those everyday stressed thoughts that niggle away at us. It asks us to put things into perspective.

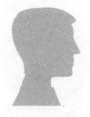

Tom worries about his general mood. He is rarely happy and sees himself as a 'glass half-empty' person. He has few friends and knows he often rubs people up the wrong way. He feels he needs to change. His stress voice says:

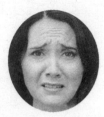

'I feel envy and hatred towards so many people. I hate myself but I don't make any moves to change. I am wasting my life.'

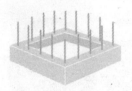

Build the foundation: stand back, pull back the blinkers, wait a minute.

Challenge

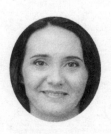

'Is life too short to think like this? When I'm on my deathbed do I want to look back on all the chances I've not taken? All the people I've snubbed? All the fears that have held me back? I'm only going to be on this earth once. I've got to confront life. I've got to give it my best shot. If things don't work out, then at least I've tried.'

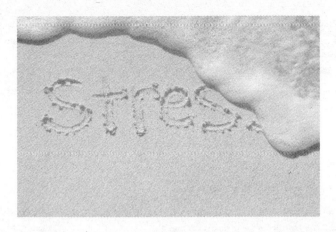

Breaking stress up

To make the Big 5 Challenges easier to deal with we need to prevent stress from getting too high in the first place.

Breaking stress up is a great skill for those of us who can see a link between stress and what is going on in our lives. So if you noticed patterns in Chapter 3, you can use this skill to prevent stress by nipping it in the bud.

Here is a crucial question: if you know you have a stressful event coming up, how do you handle the stress? Most people answer 'I'll just not think about it.' Sounds sensible, but try this:

Don't think of a skateboarding penguin.
Do not think of a skateboarding penguin.
Under no circumstances think of a skateboarding penguin.

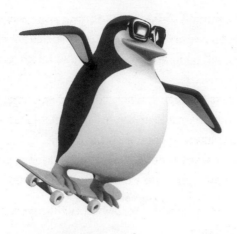

Chances are you just thought of a skateboarding penguin even though you were told not to. This is a daft trick but it makes a serious point: the more we try *not* to think about something, the more likely we are to think about it. So trying to cope with an upcoming stressful event by not thinking about it is doomed from the start.

So if *not thinking* about it is a bad idea then *thinking* about it should be a good idea. And it is – as long as you think about it in the right way. This skill gets you thinking about it while working out ways to cope with it using your common sense voice. And that is what 'breaking stress up' is all about: it breaks the stress into 'bite-size' bits. It divides into three stages:

Prepare to face the stress In Stage 1 you take control of your thoughts instead of the thoughts taking control of you. You use your common sense voice to think your way out of stress. If you *prepare* well, by the time the event comes along you will be in greater control and much more likely to cope.

Face the stress In Stage 2, when you *face* the stress, you will be much more capable of staying in control and, therefore, much more likely to cope with the event.

Review how it went When you *review*, in Stage 3, you can work out how well or how badly your plan went.

'Breaking stress up' links up well with a skill covered in Chapter 7, 'Problem Solving'.

Prepare to face the stress

Once you focus on the future event that you think will cause you problems, set up your plan for coping by working out how you can deal with it. Some helpful thoughts could be:

- I am not going to hide or run away from it.
- I can work out a plan to deal with this.
- I can expect to feel stressed – that's OK.
- I won't know how it will go until I get there. So make sure I get there.

Face the stress

Your task here is to put your plan into action, to stay focused on this plan and to use your new skills, such as relaxation. Some helpful thoughts could be:

- Take it one step at a time.
- Relax, I'm in control. Keep the breathing steady.
- I feel a bit stressed – that's normal. Just stay on top of this.
- Get the blinkers back – see the big picture.

Review how it went

Having *prepared to face the stress* and having *faced the stress*, it is time to see how well or badly your plan worked; to see if you could improve it for next time and to pat yourself on the back for going through with it. Some helpful thoughts could be:

- Well done. I could have got out of it but I faced the fear.
- I had to leave – so it did not work – what can I learn from this?
- I've taken a step forward – I'm getting there, slowly but surely.
- I coped because I worked at it – practice makes perfect.

You might want to use a practice form like the one below.

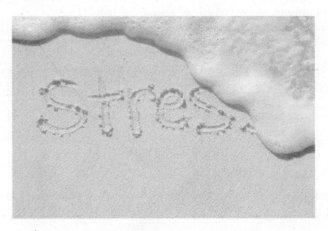

Breaking up stress practice form

Preparing
Facing up
Reviewing

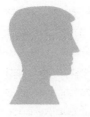 Ray's mother has asked him to come to a family get-together on Saturday evening. Ray hates these nights and gets stressed thinking about being with some members of the family he doesn't get on well with. As a way of coping, he tends to avoid going. If he does go, he tends to drink too much, gets easily annoyed and, sometimes, ends up spoiling the night for his mother. However, she really wants him to come as long as he behaves. He feels obliged to go. This is what he says:

> 'I really can't handle this. I get too uptight and I find it so hard to cope with my sister and her husband. They know what buttons to push and they wind me up. I need a few beers to give me the courage to go, but once I've had a few more I look for arguments and create an atmosphere. But my old mum has told me I have to go and I don't want to upset her – upset her by not going, or upset her by going and being a pain in the backside. So I guess I just have to do it. But as I get too stressed thinking about it, I'll just not think about it till the day itself.'

Ray decides against avoiding and, instead, will go to his mother's house. So he is going to face his fears. Good plan. But he decides 'I'll just not think about it.' Bad plan. The more he tries *not* to think of something, the more likely he is to think of it. So trying to put this stressful event to the back of his mind won't work. His stress voice will just get louder and louder and the stress will get stronger and stronger. Thinking about it and working out ways to deal with it makes a lot more sense and will give Ray a much better chance of coping on the night.

So, on Sunday, Ray becomes aware of the stressed thoughts about the get-together the following Saturday. He still decides to 'just not think about it' on Monday and Tuesday. But as you can see, the stress voice slowly gets louder and louder and less and less controllable as the week goes on. As he reaches his mother's door, his stress level is so high that his chances of coping once inside are poor. His sister just has to look at him . . .

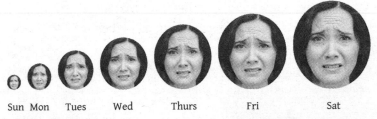

Sun Mon   Tues   Wed   Thurs   Fri   Sat

So 'I'll just not think about it' isn't a great coping skill. Waiting until he is at his mother's house to try to control his stress is also not a good coping skill. It just makes the task so much harder. Much better to *prepare* to face the stress as soon as he can. So Ray should challenge the thoughts the second they appear. This is what should happen:

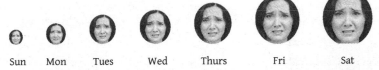

Sun   Mon   Tues   Wed   Thurs   Fri   Sat

Ray's stressed voice is still there and it does get a bit louder (stress always increases the closer we get to the event we dread). But by thinking about how to handle the night using his common sense voice, he stays much calmer. So reaching his mother's door, he is more in control – it will take a lot more to get him to lose it once inside.

So, in the second stage, he continues to use his common sense voice to talk himself through the night as he *faces the stress*.

Once the night is over it is tempting for Ray to go home, pour himself a big drink and try to put the night out of his mind. Having the drink is fine but, as he has made a plan and carried it out, it is crucial that he *reviews* how it went. So the final stage is to consider if the plan worked, how well it worked or, if it didn't work, why not? In reviewing, failure isn't all bad. Ray can learn from it and be better next time.

On the next page, you can see the kind of statements Ray used *before* (preparing), *during* (facing) and *after* (reviewing).

Prepare to face the stress

Once you focus on the future event that you think will cause you stress, you set up your plan for coping by thinking how you can deal with it.

- I can work out a plan to deal with coping with my sister.
- I can expect to feel stressed – that's OK – accept it.
- I won't know how it will go until I get there. So make sure I get there.
- I don't have to enjoy myself. I just have to cope.

Face the stress

Your task here is to put your plan into action, to stay focused on this plan and to use your new skills, such as relaxation. Some helpful thoughts could be:

- Take it one step at a time.
- I feel a bit stressed – that's normal.
- Relax, I'm in control. Keep the breathing sorted.
- Don't sulk in the corner, help Mum, talk to my sister about her holiday.

Review how it went

Having prepared to face the stress and having faced the stress, it is time to see how well or badly your plan worked, to see if you could improve it for next time and to pat yourself on the back for going through with it. Some helpful thoughts could be:

- Well done. I could have got out of it but I faced up to it.
- I had to leave – so it did not work – what can I learn from this?
- I've taken a step forward – I'm getting there, slowly but surely.
- Didn't like being there but Mum was pleased with me – job done!

Combining your skills

Ray could make sure he keeps his caffeine levels low on the day. He could use breathing retraining as he walks to his mother's house. He could make sure he stops his muscles tensing in the house.

Ray could use the Big 5 Challenges (three of them fit very well here):

'**What is the worst thing that can happen if I go?** I'll argue with my sister again. I did that before and yet my mum sticks by me and, in fairness to sis, she still talks to me. I could be uptight and unhappy. I don't want that to happen, but it's hardly the end of the world.'

'**Am I right to think that I can't cope with a get-together?** Sometimes it is OK – never a good night, but OK. Accept that we are never going to be close, but at least we can get on. And I love my old mum to bits and hate letting her down. It would be great to get to the end of the night and Mum thanks me for coming and behaving myself! I'd be so pleased if I can do that for her.'

'**Is life too short to feel like this?** I feel at my lowest ebb in years. Having family support does help, and maybe if I'm nicer to my sister she'll be nicer to me. I'm sure it isn't fun for her either.'

Last words

The aim of Chapter 6 is to help you challenge your thoughts and to nip stress in the bud. Controlling thoughts is hard work. But it is crucial, and is a major step in controlling your stress. So we will come back to these skills later and see how you can combine them with the others you will learn as you work your way through this book.

The positive circle is beginning to gain strength. Chapter 7 builds on this by teaching you how to control your actions. You might start to see how all the skills come together and help you to see the big picture.

7

Controlling your actions

In this chapter we focus on facing your fears, stepping out of your comfort zone and problem solving. We will also look at bringing all the skills together.

Part 1 Information

We all know how much stress can affect our actions: we avoid doing things or going places in case we can't cope; we can't sit still; we get into arguments over silly things; we withdraw rather than risk being overwhelmed.

Actions like these badly affect our self-confidence and our self-esteem. We put on the blinkers and start to grasshopper think. Our hearts race, we sweat, our muscles tense. But don't be disheartened: the more skills we learn, the weaker our vicious circle becomes.

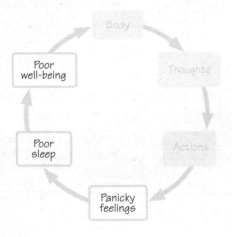

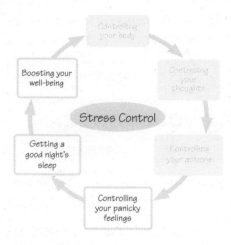

This chapter teaches skills that will change our actions and, as a result, lower our stress and give our confidence and self-esteem the chance to grow. We will see that controlling our actions helps to feed our positive circle:

There are two main actions to consider: **avoidance** and **behaviour**.

Avoidance

Our actions in this respect are not always black and white: we might feel able to talk to some people but not others; drive on certain roads at certain times but avoid others; be able to go to a particular place sometimes but not other times, and so on. Think back to Chapter 5 – avoidance is based on *flight* – the instinct to run away because we feel threatened.

We should also bear in mind *escape* – the close cousin of avoidance – which happens when we go into a situation but always have one eye on the exit. A common example is when we go to the cinema but sit at the end of the back row 'just in case'. Although this may seem common sense, we will see why this action helps keep stress alive when we look at 'stepping out of your comfort zone' later.

Some of the common things we may avoid when stressed are listed below:

Making decisions	Taking responsibility
Talking to neighbours	Driving
Shopping	Reading about illness
Social life	Being alone
Dealing with bills, etc.	Expressing opinions
Being far from home	Using public transport

Just about everyone in the world takes evasive action in an attempt to avoid stress: it's probably the most common way of coping. And there is an obvious reason for this – it is a superb way to reduce stress quickly. But it is not the answer.

Vinay's story

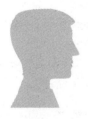

Sarah is leaving the office to go to a new job. A leaving do has been arranged and all the staff are expected to go. The plan is to meet in the pub for a few drinks, get something to eat and then the younger ones will head to a club. Vinay will be expected to do all three.

He gets on well with Sarah and knows she will be hurt if he does not go. But Vinay gets very stressed coping with events such as this. The club in particular seems very daunting.

He finds himself getting more and more uptight during the day at work. The others are excited about the night and this makes him worse. His heart is racing, his hands are a little shaky and he feels a bit sick. The 'what ifs' are strong: 'What if I make a fool of myself?'; 'What if I can't talk in the restaurant?'; 'What if everyone is drunk and makes a fool of me?'

Vinay feels overwhelmed. He plans an escape route. He tells Sarah that he is feeling unwell and, although he really wants to go, he might not make it. He has the feeling Sarah knows he is making his excuses.

Vinay goes home and, as the time to get ready and set off for the pub gets closer, his stress level increases. He feels overwhelmed and decides he can't go. He texts Sarah to say he is unwell.

In a flash, his stress level drops. Avoidance has worked. But . . .

Two hours later Vinay is at home, thinking of his friends in the pub having a great time, making it a special night for Sarah, talking about why he isn't there. He is angry with himself:

> 'I've let Sarah down. I could have coped with it. They are a good bunch of guys. I've let them all down. What's wrong with me? Why can't I cope the way they all can? It will be awful going into work tomorrow. I'm a complete failure. I hate myself.'

And his stress level has just got worse. Remember:

Avoidance works well in the short term but, in the long run, makes us worse.

The answer to Vinay's problems is 'face your fears'. Later on we will see how he did this, aided by the other skills he had learned in stress control.

Behaviour

This is about how we act when we get stressed.

Some common ways our behaviour is affected by stress

Anger outbursts	Take longer to do things
Make more mistakes	Drink, smoke or use drugs more
Cry	Argue
Always rushed	Take more risks
Accident prone	Do too many things at the one time
Check more	Go quiet
Withdrawn	Easily distracted
Can't sit at peace	Stammer
Speak too fast	Speak too quietly
Bite your nails	Disorganized

When our behaviour changes:

- We may become more self-conscious.
- It can affect others as they see our stressed actions.
- We see it as a sign that we are not coping.

And, just like avoidance, this lowers our self-esteem and self-confidence and keeps our stress alive.

Part 2 Controlling your actions – *skills*

Facing your fears

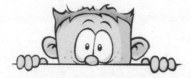

Stepping out of your comfort zone

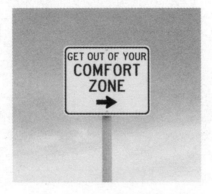

Problem solving

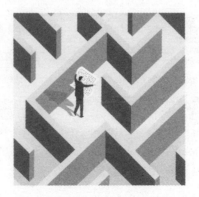

You will also see how to combine these with the skills you have learned in the earlier chapters.

Facing your fears

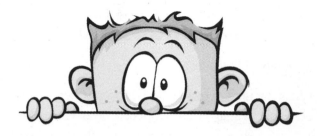

Avoidance is probably the most common way we try to cope with stress and that is because it works – the second we decide to avoid going somewhere or doing something that we think will cause us stress, we feel much better. However, as previously stated, while avoidance works well in the short term, it makes us worse in the long term.

And this is because when we avoid:

- We tell ourselves we can't cope.
- We see threats all the time.
- We measure life by what we can't do rather than by what we can.

This lowers our self-esteem and self-confidence and keeps our stress alive. So how do we change this? Well, the answer to the question has been known for hundreds of years: what do you do if you fall off a horse? You get back on it because, if you don't, the chance of getting back on any horse in the future gets less and less likely.

Of all the laws of psychology, this one will always remain true:

Facing our fears often makes us worse in the short term but, in the long term, makes us better.

Test the reality

If you avoid facing the things that cause you stress, you never find out what would have happened or if you could have coped. So your stress stays in place or even gets worse. If you face your fear, you can test the reality of the fear. If the thing you fear does not happen, then you can let the fear go. Even if the thing you fear does happen, is it as bad as you thought it would be? The chances are that it is not.

It is easy to tell someone to face their fears; it is far from easy to do. So the first stage is to move from saying 'I can't even look at this' to 'OK, let's take a peek at this scary thing.'

Face your fears in five stages

Stage 1 What is the fear to face?

Work out your list of the things you avoid and need to face up to.

Stage 2 What do I think will happen when I face my fear?

Try to predict what will happen. Use the 'controlling your thoughts' skills ('What is the worst thing can that happen?' is good for this). Once you have faced the fear, see how good this prediction was.

Stage 3 Work out a plan

Make sure you use all the skills you have already learned, e.g. relaxation and breaking stress up.

Stage 4 Put it into action

Face your fear.

Stage 5 Review

Did it work? If not, why not? Can you now go on and tackle other fears?

Note that Stages 3, 4 and 5 are the same as with breaking stress up in Chapter 6 (preparing, facing up and reviewing). You might find the practice form below useful.

Facing your fears practice form

1 What is the fear to face?
2 What do I think will happen when I face my fear?
3 Work out a plan: preparing
4 Put it into action
5 Reviewing

Stepping out of your comfort zone

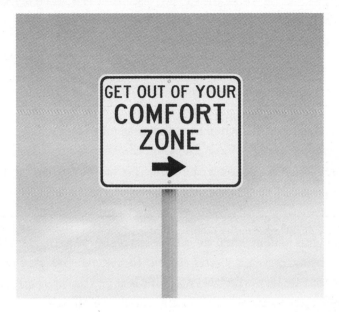

We have learned that facing your fear always works in the long run. However, some people say they do face their fear, again and again, but the fear never breaks down. Why is this?

It turns out that, while they are in a stressful situation (facing their fear), they do something as a way to protect themselves. This is to try to limit how bad they feel while facing their fear. This sabotages their good work because it stops them from *truly* facing their fear. What they do helps in the short term but makes them worse in the long run.

In other words, they play safe by staying in their comfort zone. To get over the stress, they need to step out of it and truly face their fear. Staying in the comfort zone can be very subtle and hard to spot. Let us look at how Liz and Sean do it.

Liz has suffered from panic attacks on and off for four years. She reckons she has had well over 100 attacks. Each time the panic hits, she has this scary thought: 'I'm going to faint.' Liz bravely tries to face her fear and goes into all the places she feels more at risk – busy shops, social clubs, football matches. Yet she doesn't get over the panic. Liz has never fainted in a panic, so why doesn't she lose the fear after more than 100 false alarms?

Sean gets uptight when he is on a bus on his own. He fears the bus being crowded, being unable to get out and unable to breathe. He knows he has to face his fear and travel by bus. But week after week he still has the same level of distress, even though he seems to be facing his fear. He is about to give up trying as he is getting nowhere. Nothing too bad has happened to him, so why doesn't Sean lose the fear after so many bus trips?

The reason Liz doesn't get over the fear is because she does something to try to protect herself and lessen her sense of threat. The second she has the thought and starts to feel light-headed, she either sits down or leans against something as she thinks she will be less likely to faint. This makes sense to her at the time; after all, who wants to faint?

The reason Sean doesn't get over the fear is because he does something to try to protect himself and lessen his sense of threat. As soon as he gets on the bus, he starts texting friends and family, tells them he is on the bus and asks them to keep texting as he is uptight. They text back and forth for the duration of the bus journey. This helps keep Sean distracted and, he believes, allows him to survive the journey.

On the face of it, what Liz and Sean do seems to make sense. But we are back to the big message learned in Chapter 2: what helps in the short term may actually make you worse in the long term.

False friends

These simple actions – sitting/leaning and texting – are false friends: they seem to be helping but, in fact, they sabotage all the hard work and courage Liz and Sean show in trying to face their fears, and further reduce their confidence levels.

The problem is that doing these things feeds the sense of threat. Liz and Sean are telling themselves that they *need* to protect themselves, and that the threat is real. They feel playing safe is the last line of defence. But if they had not played safe, they could have tested the reality of their fears.

Liz bravely goes into the places she fears. Afterwards, instead of praising herself and patting herself on the back, she says, 'Thank goodness I sat down there. Otherwise I would have fainted.' She has convinced herself that the next time she feels faint she should sit down as fast as she can.

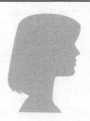

She has not tested the reality of her fear – would she have fainted had she not sat down? She can't answer that because she has stayed in her comfort zone. She needs to step out her comfort zone and test the reality of her beliefs.

To do that, the next time the panic hits she has to stand her ground. Now she can test the reality of her fear. Two things can happen: either she will faint or she won't.

She hasn't fainted in her last 100 or so panics. So the odds are good that she won't faint next time. And if she doesn't then she has truly faced her fear and found it wanting. Now she can begin to believe she can cope, pat herself on the back and start to build up her self-confidence.

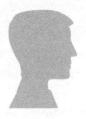 Sean has been bravely going on buses for the last two months and it is not getting any easier. He is about to give up. He gets off the bus and says to himself, 'Thank goodness I was able to keep texting with my mates. Otherwise I'm sure I wouldn't have coped.' He will believe that texting is the best way to cope on the bus and will do it next time. In fact, he would not step on the bus if he had left his phone at home.

He has not tested the reality of his fear – would he have been overwhelmed if he hadn't texted? He can't answer that because he stays in his comfort zone. He needs to step out his comfort zone and test the reality of his beliefs.

To do that, the next time he gets on a bus, he has to keep his phone in his pocket and see what happens. He can now test the reality of his fear. Two things can happen: either he will be overwhelmed or he won't. He will likely be more stressed (but he has many more skills up his sleeve that he can use now – challenging his thinking, etc.).

The odds are good that things won't be as bad as he thinks. And if he doesn't text then he has truly faced his fear and found it wanting. Now he can begin to believe he can cope, pat himself on the back and start to build up his self-confidence.

Facing the fear

Both Liz and Sean, by stepping out of their comfort zones, can now truly face their fear. Instead of giving the credit to their 'false friends' they can take the credit themselves: 'I coped because I faced my fears and while it made me more stressed in the short term, in the long term I felt a lot better.' Only now will Liz and Sean start to get on top of their stress.

Here are some common things people do to stay in their comfort zone.

Try to focus your mind on certain thoughts or images to stop your mind spiralling out of control.
Rehearse what you are going to say at a social event (as you fear making a fool of yourself).
Avoid answering the phone or door at home.
Look busy to avoid having to talk to others.
Walk through the shops with your eyes to the ground to prevent meeting someone you know.
Rely on alcohol to cope with an event.
Always agree with others.
Hide your face with your hair (as you fear others will see you blush).

Carry a bottle of water with you to keep you cool and your mouth moist.
Play with your phone in a café when you are on your own.
Pretend to be writing notes in a meeting (as you fear coming across badly if you have to talk).
Have a range of excuses ready for having a red face: 'It's so hot in here', 'I'm not well' (as you fear others will notice and think badly of you).
Make sure you carry your mobile in case you need to call for help.

We can learn how to step out of our comfort zone in five stages. Note that Stages 3, 4 and 5 are the same as for Facing Your Fears above, and Breaking Stress Up in Chapter 6.

Step out of your comfort zone in five stages

Stage 1 How do you try to stay in your comfort zone? What 'props' do you use? Decide how much they help or hinder you

Write down all the things you do or think to try to stop something bad happening to you. You should also think of anything you use to help ('props'), e.g. some people keep a diazepam tablet in their pocket all the time.

Stage 2 Predict what would happen if you stepped out of your comfort zone

Run the scene right to the end. If you did not try to play safe, what would happen? ('What is the worst thing that would happen?' is very good for this.) Have there been times when you didn't play safe? What happened?

Stage 3 Work out a plan ('preparing')

Work out what you want to tackle and plan how to step out of your comfort zone. To make this easier, combine the skills learned so far, e.g. controlling your body and controlling your thoughts. Then do it.

Stage 4 Facing up

Do it.

Stage 5 Review

How did it go? Was it better or worse than you predicted? Why was this? Do you need to change your plan for the next time?

Keep going until you have completely stepped out of your comfort zone and left all the ways you try to protect yourself far behind. You are now facing your fear and, in doing so, breaking down your stress. It is hard work, but well worth it in the end.

You might want to use the practice form below.

Stepping out of your comfort zone practice form

1 How do you try to stay in your comfort zone?
2 Predict what would happen if you stepped out of your comfort zone
3 Work out a plan: preparing
4 Facing up: do it
5 Reviewing

Problem solving

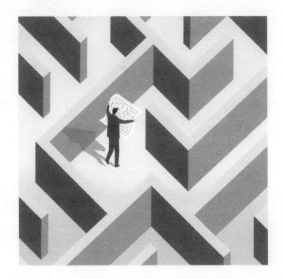

This is a great way to help you deal with any problem in your life.

- You take on problems one at a time.
- You break each problem into eight 'bite-size' stages.
- As you pick up this skill, you gain a greater sense of control in your life and your self-confidence and self-esteem get a chance to build.

The stages are:

Controlling your actions

STAGE 1	Clearly state the problem

STAGE 2	What if I don't solve the problem?

STAGE 3	What if I *do* solve the problem?

STAGE 4	Brainstorm

STAGE 5	Choose the best option

STAGE 6	Work out a plan

STAGE 7	Put it into action

STAGE 8	Review

Note that Stages 6, 7 and 8 below are the same as for Breaking Stress Up, Facing Your Fear and Stepping Out of Your Comfort Zone.

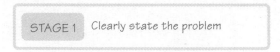

STAGE 1   Clearly state the problem

Bad examples

'This house gets me down.'
'I'm so bad-tempered.'

These are not clear-cut – what is it about the house? Is the mortgage or rent too high, or is it the neighbours? Is it too small? Is it too far from where you work? Are you always bad-tempered? Or only with some people or in some places?

Good examples

'The dampness in the back room is getting worse.'
'My son has no time for me now.'
Much more clear-cut. You have clearly stated the problem.

STAGE 2   What if I don't solve the problem?

If the answer is 'nothing much', then it isn't worth trying to solve it. But if you decide that your stress will go on, then move to the next stage.

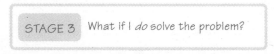

STAGE 3   What if I *do* solve the problem?

This is a much more positive question. If the answer is that your life will be improved, keep going.

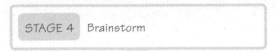

STAGE 4   Brainstorm

Try to come up with as many solutions as you can. This is a way to stretch your mind, so it doesn't matter how good or bad they are. The more you can think of, the better the chances are of finding a good one. So write down all your options.

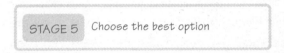

STAGE 5   Choose the best option

Go through your options one at a time and write down the pros and cons of each. Then decide which ones to keep and which to reject. You can keep as many or as few as you want, as it may take more than one option to lead to success.

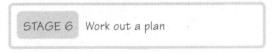

STAGE 6   Work out a plan

Work out how you are going to tackle the problem (preparing).

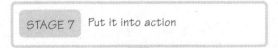

STAGE 7   Put it into action

Do it (facing up).

> STAGE 8   *Review*

Did it work?

- If it did not, why not?
- What did you learn?
- Can you improve it to make it work?
- What is the next problem you can tackle?

At the start, it can be helpful to focus on a small problem on which to practise. Once you get good at it, tackle the bigger problems that, if solved, will make your life a lot better. Then think about using problem solving to tackle some of the biggest questions in your life:

- How is your life going?
- Are you living the life you want?
- Are you living up to your ideals?
- Are you making a go of it?

Once you get good at problem solving you should be able to do it in your head. At this stage, however, it is a lot easier to write down the eight stages. Use the practice form below to help.

Problem solving practice form

| STAGE 1 | Clearly state the problem |

| STAGE 2 | What if I don't solve the problem? |

| STAGE 3 | What if I *do* solve the problem? |

| STAGE 4 | Brainstorm |

| STAGE 5 | Choose the best option |

| STAGE 6 | Work out a plan |

| STAGE 7 | Put it into action |

| STAGE 8 | Review |

Sam's problem

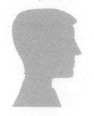

Sam has had problems with low mood since childhood. He describes himself as someone who struggles to be positive in life, and has always regarded himself as a failure and a loser. Sam believes he is the way he is because of his father who, Sam feels, never showed him any love and rarely spent time with him. Sam grew up believing that if his dad didn't think anything of him, why should anyone else?

He tried to stay out of his father's way, partly due to the latter's temper and partly because he assumed his dad didn't want Sam near him. Sam feels his life has been blighted and, although he still talks to his dad, he is not close. He swore when his own son was born that he would be a better father to John than his father was to him.

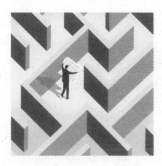

John is now nine and Sam believes he tries to keep out of Sam's way. He worries that he has failed as a father and, as a result, John will grow up with the same problems he has. Sam sees history repeating itself and feels very guilty. He decides to try problem solving:

Stage 1 Clearly state the problem

'My son has no time for me now.'

Stage 2 What if I don't solve the problem?

'It will be the same as me and my dad. I used to think he was the greatest. I ended up hating him. He was never there to help me when things were bad. I couldn't share the good times with him either. I believed he thought I was no use. I can't let that happen with my son.'

Stage 3 What if I *do* solve the problem?

'I feel so guilty that I am not the father I dearly want to be. This guilt sits heavily on me. If I thought I was doing the right thing by my son, I might get rid of some of the guilt. I would think I was a better person than I am now. My wife might gain some respect for me (I doubt she has much just now). This would help us both.'

Note that we start to see other things going on in Sam's life – it looks like he has a poor relationship with his wife. This is important. We will see in Chapter 10 why having good life support is vital in controlling stress.

Stage 4 Brainstorm

Options:

- I was the same with Dad when I was John's age. Just leave him. He will come round.
- I'll buy him a TV for his room.
- I'm so wrapped up in my problems, I've not spent any time with him for ages. We used to do a lot in the past. I could change this.
- We all eat in front of the TV. We could all sit round the table again and talk.
- My wife says I'm like a bear with a sore head. I just shout at him all the time. No wonder he steers clear of me.
- I'll ask my wife if she has any ideas. John talks to her.

Some of these options look better than others. So the next stage is for Sam to go through each one, look at the pros and cons, keep the good ones and ditch the poor ones.

Stage 5 Choose the best option

Option	Pros	Cons	Will it work?
Just leave him: he will come round	I still talk to my dad now.	I still resent my dad for not trying harder with me. I swore when John was born that I would not be like that with him.	No. Ditch it.
Buy him a TV	He wants a TV in his room.	You can't buy love.	No. Ditch it.

I could spend more time with him	He loves fishing. We could go to the river on Saturdays. I could pick him up from Cubs on Tuesdays. I could just ask him how his day was – I don't even do that.	It sounds good but will I do it? But if this worked, it would help both of us. If I felt him come round to me, I would feel less of a failure.	Yes. Don't aim too high though. Take it one step at a time.
Eat our meal at the table	We could all talk. We are like ships in the night just now. It would help keep the family strong.	None. This is good.	Yes. I know my wife wants to do this.
Stop shouting all the time	This would be great.	I try not to but I can't stop it. So I have to work at it. Use the stuff on controlling my thoughts. Try to relax more. Work out why I get angry.	Maybe. Don't aim too high though.
Ask my wife	She has just about given up on me as I don't try with John. This would show her I am trying. She might know some good ways to help me with him.	None. This is good.	Yes. I think she will help me all the way if she feels I am trying.

Sam decides to ditch Options 1 and 2, work on Options 3, 4 and 6 and keep Option 5 on the backburner. He knows Option 5 is important but feels it is beyond him at this time.

Stage 6 Work out a plan

Sam started with Option 6. He used what his wife told him to help plan Option 3.

> 'My wife asked John if he would like to go fishing. He was really keen and said he missed going with his dad. That gives me the courage to do it. I'll speak to him after our meal tonight. We'll get the rods out to check them. I will meet him from school on Friday and go to the tackle shop for a few things. We can pack up the gear as well. The two of us will do all this together.

> 'My friend will pick us up first thing. I've told him what I am trying to do and he knows I will find this stressful. But he is good at keeping me calm. He will bring his own son and he gets on well with my boy. We will be quiet when we fish so that is less pressure on me. I will not expect it to be perfect but we will do it again the next Saturday I am off if he wants to. I'll listen to relaxation exercises on my iPod to relax in the morning. I will not drink the night before as that gets me more uptight the next day.'

Stage 7 Put it into action

Do it.

Stage 8 Review

Here is Sam's review, written that night:

> 'It has rained all day and we didn't catch a thing. That put a bit of a dampener on things. I spent too much time talking to my mate and not enough to John. I shouted at him for spilling the bait. I should not have done that. He is only a young lad. It is only bait. These were the bad things. I can learn from this and not make the same mistakes next time.
>
> But, on the plus side, John said he had a good time. He wanted to know if we could do it again. I think he was wary of asking me in case I got angry or something. But I said yes and I told him I had a good time being with him (and so I did).
>
> 'My wife was pleased, but she wants to see signs that I will keep it up. Fair enough. On the whole, I'm pleased with how it went. I've taken a step forward.'

Sam, possibly without realizing it, is using other skills learned from this book. The first paragraph is all about the things that went wrong. If he keeps the blinkers on, the day will be seen as a failure. But he pulls the blinkers back and sees the good things that happened by using a form of the 'Am I right to think that . . .' challenge and ends up with a 'shades of grey' view.

It is now a regular trip. Sam still shouts a lot in the house but at least he often talks freely with and plays with his son. He feels, at long last, that he is closer to being the dad he wants to be. This helps his self-esteem and reduces his feelings of guilt. His wife sees him trying and she is slowly coming round to him again. So his relationships can improve. This will strengthen his sense of well-being (see Chapter 10). He still uses problem solving to keep on top of things.

Combining the skills

First steps, controlling your body, controlling your thoughts and, now, controlling your actions, have taught you some great skills. Each, on its own, is helpful. But it is when they are combined that they can do most to control stress. We are now ready to do this. Let's look at a real-life example which starts off with 'facing your fear' and goes on to incorporate some of the other skills covered in this book.

Vinay's story

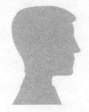

Earlier on, we looked at Vinay's story. In that scenario, he decided to avoid going to his friend's leaving do as he felt overwhelmed at the prospect of meeting up in the pub, going for a meal and then on to a club. He felt so guilty as he knew Sarah would be upset that he was not there.

What would happen if Vinay decided to test out the new skills he has acquired?

Vinay decides he has to face his fear. This is how he went about it, starting with a review of his background skills:

Exercise Since moving from another town last year, Vinay hasn't been playing five-a-side football and he isn't as fit as he feels he should be. He has started going out for short runs most nights and, after two months, is feeling better as a result. However, he realizes he likes being around others when he exercises so plans to look for a five-a-side team.

Alcohol Vinay is a social drinker and doesn't need to cut down. He rarely takes drugs.

Calm breathing (see Chapter 4) Vinay prefers this to belly breathing and uses it most days.

Caffeine He has been cutting down for a few weeks now and does feel less restless and his stomach is a lot better.

Breaking stress up: preparing

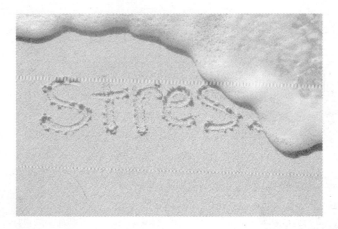

Vinay's usual approach would be to try to put a stressful event out of his mind until he has to deal with it ('Don't think of a skateboarding penguin'). He now sees that this is not a good idea and so thinks about how to handle the night out for at least one week before the date. As he *prepares* to face the stress, his coping statements, using his common sense voice, are:

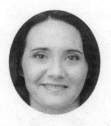

'Stop predicting how bad it will be. I won't know until I get there.'

'I've been on nights out before. I don't enjoy them but I cope OK.'

'I like most of the people I work with. And they like me. They don't give me a hard time.'

He plans to use the quick relaxation technique on the bus on the way into town. He will use the calm breathing technique as well. He plans to get in early to give him time to relax before the pub gets too busy.

Building the Foundation

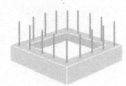

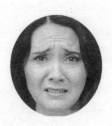

He knows he is prone to grasshopper thinking ('What if I make a fool of myself?'; 'What if I can't talk in the restaurant?'; 'What if everyone is drunk and they make a fool of me?' 'Why can't I cope the way they all can? I'm such an idiot. I hate myself.').

So he knows to **stand back, pull back the blinkers, wait a minute** to see the big picture . . . and challenge . . .

The Big 5 Challenge

He now uses the Court Case challenge and makes sure he is able to listen to his common sense voice and ignore his stressed voice.

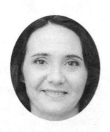

'Am I right to think I can't cope? On the one hand, I'm pretty shy. I do get tongue-tied; I can't talk as well as many of the others. But on the other hand, they all seem to like me and I like them. They've been out with me before and they are genuine about wanting me to come out again. So I must be OK. Some of the others are pretty shy too and no one holds that against them. I'm not responsible for keeping the chat going. I do feel worse at the start of the night but maybe that is normal. All of us tend to be chattier later on after a few drinks. And if I don't want to go to the club then I don't have to. It isn't a big deal.'

Stepping out of his comfort zone

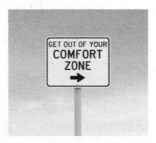

Vinay is aware that he often stays close to his friend Abby, and tries to sit beside her at the end of the table as he feels relaxed with her. He sees this as staying in his comfort zone so decides instead to sit right in the middle and 'see what happens'. He won't drink too much as this does not help his nerves.

He planned to use an excuse to avoid going on to the club – having to meet an old friend for a drink. He will not do so. He will decide later whether to go to the club or not and, if not, will tell people he simply doesn't want to go. He knows this means he is truly facing his fear so he will be more uptight at the start. This is taken into account in his *facing up* statements:

Breaking up: facing up

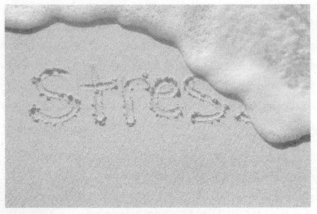

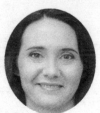

'I'm feeling pretty uptight. That's normal. Live with it. It will pass.'

'Don't drink to give myself Dutch courage. I'm the one who'll handle this.'

'Keep talking to people on my left, right and opposite. But don't jabber like a parrot.'

Breaking stress up: reviewing

Here is Vinay's review, written the next morning:

> 'Not bad. I was very uptight going into the pub. The breathing helped. The stress did come down a bit, but not much. Surprised myself by talking to people I don't know that well instead of just Abby. Tom actually told me he was uptight. Didn't guess – he always looks solid. Should have told him I was uptight too. Restaurant had some tricky moments but I coped. No appetite due to nerves and lost it a bit when I stopped thinking my way through it. Caught hold of this and felt a bit more in control. Felt tempted to make an excuse to go but didn't. Had a few more beers than planned but I was fine. Went to the club and stayed one hour. Sarah was really happy I stayed, and danced with her before I left. I'll miss her a lot. I didn't enjoy the night but I coped and that was the goal so big pat on the back. There is light at the end of the tunnel!'

Vinay left nothing to chance – he already had his background skills in place. He prepared well, he truly faced his fear having stepped out of his comfort zone, and stayed on top of his stress by thinking things through to the end. His goal was simply to cope so he achieved that. His self-confidence and self-esteem got a chance to grow, and the next time it will be that bit easier. Vinay has become his own therapist.

Last words

The aim of this chapter is to help you challenge your actions and build up your self-confidence. You should now look for ways to combine these skills with the ones you have learned in the previous chapters.

We now move on to look at skills to tackle some of the common problems often found in stress. Chapter 8 teaches you how to control panicky feelings.

8

Controlling your panicky feelings

Not everyone who has stress gets panic attacks, but most people who experience stress will have panicky feelings at some time or another. This chapter aims to teach skills that will help control these feelings and, as a result, lower stress. And, as we have seen throughout this book, this will further weaken the vicious circle.

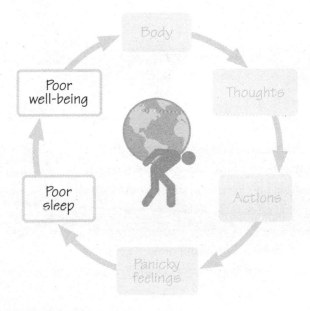

At the same time, our confidence and self-esteem get a chance to grow. Controlling panicky feelings helps to feed our positive circle:

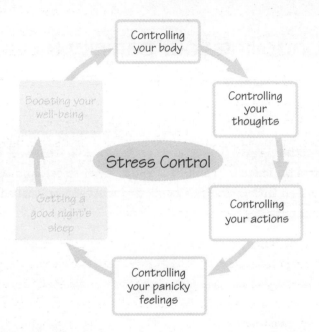

Part 1 Information

'I can be soaked in sweat in seconds and my head spins. I think my heart is going to burst out my chest. I can shake from head to toe and I often feel I need to get to a toilet. I get this surge of energy through my body. That frightens the hell out of me. I get these pins and needles in my fingers and arms and I feel like I can't get a proper breath.'

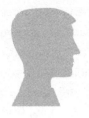

'I get so panicky for no reason and my mind goes to mush – I can't think sensibly to save myself. It's like everything speeds up so fast and I just kind of lose it. I'm always amazed (and scared) by the way my body reacts in seconds. I suppose it's the feeling that I'm losing control.'

The word 'panic' is derived from the Greek god, Pan, whose name gave rise to the Greek word *panikon*, meaning 'sudden fear'. Pan would lie in wait for people in remote mountain passes, jump out at them as they passed and scare them to death. Hence 'panic' means being in a state of terror.

Note that although they cause great stress, panicky feelings are not in themselves dangerous.

When you first experience panicky feelings, you may feel you are going mad. You may call your GP. You may rush to hospital in fear that you are having a heart attack or stroke (see the box below for more details). Panicky feelings can last from a few seconds to a few hours and may leave you feeling shaken, tense and exhausted. You may find that your life increasingly revolves around trying to stop the next panic.

Let's look at panicky feelings in terms of thoughts, actions and body.

Panic and heart attacks

As some of the signs of a panic attack are similar to those of a heart attack, e.g. chest pain, you can see why people can mistake one for the other. (Find out more about the symptoms of a heart attack on the webpage of the British Heart Foundation www.bhf.org.uk/doubtkills.) If you suffer from frequent or long-lasting chest pain, it is wise to seek medical advice. If you have a good reason to believe you are at risk of a heart attack, or you have any serious doubts about your chest pain, it is important to get yourself checked out. But if the doctor has recently ruled out any heart problem it is less likely that further chest pain is caused by a heart attack. The table below looks at some of the main differences.

	Heart attack	Panic attack
Pain	• May or not be present. • If present, you may have a crushing feeling (like someone standing on your chest). • This pain is usually felt in the centre of your chest and may extend to the left arm, jaw, neck and back. • Pain, if present, is not usually made worse by breathing or by pressing on the chest. • Pain, if present, is usually persistent and lasts longer than 5–10 minutes.	• Any pain is usually described as 'sharp'. • The pain tends to be felt over the heart. • Pain is usually made worse by breathing in and out and pressing on the centre of the chest. • Pain usually disappears within about 5–10 minutes.
Tingling	• Tingling, if present, is usually in the left arm.	• Tingling is usually present all over the body.

Vomiting	• Common.	• You may feel sick but vomiting is less common.
Breathing	• A heart attack does not cause you to breathe more quickly or too quickly (hyperventilation). With a heart attack, you may feel a little short of breath.	• Breathing too quickly or too deeply (hyperventilation) is a very common panic response experienced before a panic attack.

Adapted from the World Health Organisation *Guide to Mental Health in Primary Care* (2000)

Thoughts You may feel a rush of fear and feel that you are losing control. You might feel that something awful is about to happen to you, even though you may not be able to say what that might be.

Actions You may avoid going to places where you think you are more likely to feel panicky. You may avoid doing certain things for the same reason.

Body The body reacts in much the same way as it does to stressful situations. But the symptoms may be *much* stronger. Your heart rate can double in a few minutes, and that has a momentous effect on the rest of the body; it is no wonder that it can fill you with terror (the 'fear of fear').

The next pages look at common thoughts, action and body signs associated with panicky feelings.

Thoughts

I'm losing my mind.	I'm going to lose control of my bowels or bladder.
I'm having a heart attack.	I'm going to do something stupid.
I'm losing control.	They are all looking at me.
I'm going to die.	I'll never be normal again.
I'm going to pass out.	I am worried about my body state, e.g. pulse rate.
I'm going to make a fool of myself.	I'm confused.
I've got to get out of here.	I can't stand this any longer.

Actions

BEHAVIOUR	AVOIDANCE
Can't stay still	Exertion (for fear of bringing on an attack) (for example)
Fidgeting	Sex, running for a bus, sports
Foot tapping	Getting into arguments (fear of getting angry)
Snapping at people	Staying alone (no one to help you)
Pacing up and down	Being far from home
Yawning	Going abroad (too far from 'safety')
Sighing	Busy places
Gulping in breath	Enclosed places

Body

Palpitations or heart racing
Sweating
Nausea (sometimes vomiting)
Tingling or numbness, e.g. fingers and/or toes, around mouth and nose, sometimes on one side of body
Changes to vision, e.g. stars in front of eyes, blurring, tunnel vision
Breathlessness
Smothering sensation
Chest pains or tightness
Hot and/or cold flushes
Choking sensations
Cold, clammy hands
Muscle tension
Exhaustion
Shaking or trembling
Dizziness or faintness
Unreal feeling
Upset stomach

Types of panic feelings

Panic feelings you can predict

You may think that if you have once had panicky feelings in a busy pub, you will feel the same if you go back to that or any other pub. You may think that if you get angry or exert yourself you will upset your body and therefore will feel panicky.

You must face these fears if you are to get better. Use the skills learned earlier about controlling your body, thoughts and actions.

Panic feelings you can't predict

Most panic attacks seem to come out of the blue. You may feel OK; then, for no reason you can see, you start to feel panicky. Then you may become fearful since you feel you have no control. As you can't predict when panicky feelings could hit you, you don't know how to prevent the next attack. Sometimes the *fear* of feeling panicky is as bad as *being* panicky.

Night-time panic feelings

You can go to bed feeling fine, then wake up suddenly feeling panicky. These 'nocturnal panics' are more common in the first few hours of sleep. The most common signs are shortness of breath, racing heart, hot and cold flushes, a choking feeling, trembling and a fear of dying. You may fear going to sleep as a result. You may sleep with the window open as you think there is not enough air in the room. If so, you may be trying to stay in your comfort zone.

The vicious circle

Although it may feel like it, panic feelings do not actually come out of the blue. Panic feelings are a *reaction*. Once you learn about the things that trigger panicky feelings, you can take the first step in controlling them. As we have seen, your thoughts, actions and body feed each other. Let's look at how this works with regard to panic feelings.

The role of thoughts

As the feeling of panic seems to come out of nowhere, and hits you with such strength, you may think:

'This can't be stress. I'm losing control. I'm going mad.'

If you believe these thoughts you will start to feel more stress as your grasshopper leaps. The more stress you feel, the more it affects your thoughts, and also your actions.

The role of actions

Panicky feelings will affect your actions, and this will feed back into your thoughts:

'Look at the state I'm in – I'm acting like an idiot. They're all looking at me. I've got to get out of here.'

If you start to avoid going to certain places or doing certain things for fear of feeling panicky, you will also be aware that you are restricting your life out of fear. This will affect your self-confidence and self-esteem. As seen in Chapter 7 it is common practice to stay in your comfort zone in a (mistaken) attempt to feel better.

The role of the body

Feeling panicky often makes you tune into your body. This is no surprise, given the very unpleasant ways your body may react to these feelings. In turn this has a detrimental effect on your thoughts:

'I'm so dizzy. I'm going to pass out.'

'My stomach is heaving – I'm going to throw up.'

One aspect of your body's reaction stands out: breathing . . .

- When you breathe in, you breathe in **oxygen.**
- When you breathe out, you breathe out **carbon dioxide (CO2).**

When you breathe in, oxygen is taken to your lungs and is then carried round your body in the bloodstream. Oxygen is food: it feeds the millions of cells in your body. The cells eat up the oxygen, then turn it into waste – carbon dioxide (CO2) – which is pushed back into the bloodstream, into the lungs and breathed out.

The important word here is *balance*. Your rate of breathing should fit the amount of energy (or 'food') your body needs. So if you are playing football, running for a bus, digging the garden, your body needs more food in the form of oxygen. So you breathe faster and deeper – let's say twenty breaths each minute.

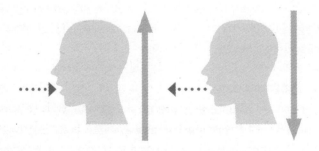

Although you might be breathing fast, the cells take up all the oxygen so all twenty breaths are converted to carbon dioxide. The oxygen and carbon dioxide in your bloodstream are therefore in balance, keeping the body nice and settled.

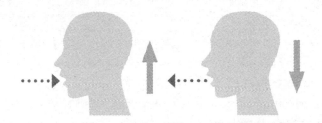

When, a few hours later, you are sitting in front of the TV at home, you only need to breathe ten times each minute as your body needs less energy. The millions of cells gobble up all these ten breaths of oxygen, convert all of it to waste and, again, the oxygen/CO_2 balance will be maintained (albeit at a much lower level), keeping your body calm.

Hyperventilation (HV)

Hyper (too much) *ventilation* (breathing) means you are breathing too fast for your needs. Once your fight/flight reaction kicks in (see Chapter 5), your body is filled with a rush of energy. As we have seen, one of the changes is that we breathe deeper and quicker and take in more oxygen. This is fine if you have to flee from danger, e.g. run from a grizzly bear, as you will use up the extra energy. One of the problems with panicky feelings is that the threats you worry about are not something you can fight or run from. So you are left filled with this extra energy (in the shape of oxygen) that you can't burn up.

As your cells don't need this food, they push much of the oxygen back into your bloodstream where it 'sticks' to your blood. So the amount of oxygen in your bloodstream rises, while your level of carbon dioxide (CO_2) drops (as the cells haven't taken up all the oxygen and so don't produce CO_2 waste). Plus, as you have to breathe out each time you breathe in, you lose more CO_2. So the amount of CO_2 in your blood-stream drops. You lose the balance – you have too much oxygen and too little CO_2 in your bloodstream. This causes two things to happen:

1 Your blood becomes more alkaline.

2 Some of your blood vessels narrow for a short time, resulting in less blood reaching the brain.

This may cause you to feel or experience:

• Dizzy;
• Faint;
• Confused;
• 'Unreal';
• Breathlessness, choking;
• Blurred vision.

It also means less blood gets to other parts of the body. This may cause:

• Raised heart rate (as it to tries to pump blood around the body);
• Numbness or tingling in fingers, feet, mouth;

- Stiff muscles;
- Clammy, cold hands.

Your body is now working hard. This may cause you to feel or experience:

- Hot, flushed and sweaty;
- Tired out;
- Aches and pains in your chest as if you have a tight belt around your ribs ('belly breathing' – see Chapter 5 – will help to ease this);
- Yawning, sighing or gulping in air (a sign of HV).

Note All these symptoms are caused by HV and not by stress. Yet they are very similar to how some people say they feel when they are panicky. So controlling the HV will help you control the symptoms. This will then help you control (or prevent) panic feelings. Do remember:

HV can be very unpleasant but it is not dangerous.

If you hyperventilate quickly – increase your breathing to, say, thirty breaths a minute – these symptoms can come on in seconds (e.g. if you get a sudden shock). It is more common to increase your breathing from, say, eleven times to twelve times a minute. This may seem no big deal, but with every minute that passes you have one extra breath of oxygen lying in your bloodstream and a similarly reduced amount of CO_2. And the signs and symptoms noted above slowly grow.

After one hour, you have sixty extra breaths and have lost sixty equivalent amounts of CO_2. The balance is slowly changing.

The body tries to cope with the slow change and you may not get any signs of the HV. But you will get to the point of no return when your CO_2 drops below a certain level and the symptoms may appear without warning. This could happen after a simple yawn (you lose a lot of CO_2 when you yawn).

It's the straw that breaks the camel's back. It seems to come out of the blue. Because you don't see why the symptoms have kicked in, you start to think that something awful is about to happen. And this leads you to feeling panicky. See how the vicious circle is created:

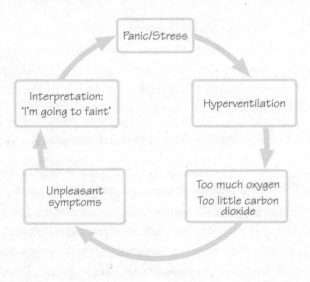

And, by combining the skills we have already learned, how the positive circle helps us get rid of panicky feelings:

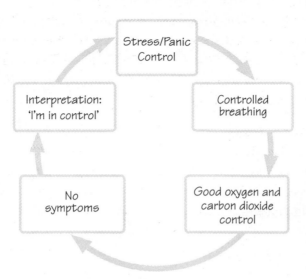

If you think you are going to faint the sense of threat is given a boost, thus increasing the stress/panicky feelings. And so the vicious circle is fed. Everyone who hyperventilates will get the same symptoms. They do not *cause* you to feel panicky; it is the way you *interpret* the symptoms that causes you to feel panicky.

This is where the panic/stress enters the circle. If, for example, you believe that you are about to have a heart attack, faint or go mad, it is common sense that you feel stressed/panicky at the thought. What is wrong in the first place is the way you have *interpreted* the symptoms. So let's take a look at the symptoms of hyperventilation.

Signs of hyperventilation

When under stress (circle Yes or No) do you:

Feel light-headed or dizzy?	YES	NO
Feel you are going to faint?	YES	NO
Yawn, sigh or gulp in air?	YES	NO
Feel short of breath?	YES	NO
Feel your breathing is shallow?	YES	NO
Feel your breathing speeds up?	YES	NO
Become aware of chest pains?	YES	NO
Get a numb or tingling feeling around the mouth and nose and/or in your fingers and toes?	YES	NO

The more times you answer 'Yes', the more likely it is that hyperventilation may be feeding your stress. This is good news, as learning to control your breathing will help you to control it. You will learn how to do this in Part 2 below.

Part 2 Controlling panicky feelings skills

Controlling your body

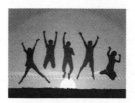

Controlling your thoughts

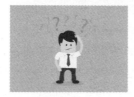

Controlling your actions

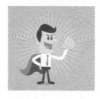

Reducing the risk of feeling panicky

Controlling your body

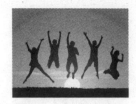

Controlling your body

When you hyperventilate you may feel that you do not have *enough* air in your lungs. As we have seen, you actually have *too much*. You have to fight against the desire to take deep breaths as this will make things worse – it just floods the bloodstream with more oxygen. Keep a grip on your breathing. If you are prone to HV, check every ten minutes that your breathing is nice and slow (about ten to twelve breaths a minute suits many of us), until you get into the habit of breathing at the right rate for you. A good way to keep your body calm is to use the skills you have already learned (choose the one that suits you best).

Calm breathing
- Breathe in slowly through your nose for a count of three to four seconds.
- Hold this for three to four seconds and breathe out through your mouth over a count of six to eight seconds.
- Repeat this three times.
- Do this each hour.

Belly breathing

Sit in a comfy chair and relax as much as you can.

- Take a slow normal breath (not a deep breath) and think '*1*' to yourself.
- As you breathe out, think '*relax*'; breathe in again and think '*2*'; breathe out and think '*relax*'.
- Keep doing this up to *10*. When you reach *10*, reverse and start back down to *1*.

Try to put everything else out of your mind. It may help to see the numbers and the word 'relax' in your mind's eye (try this at www.stresscontrolaudio.com).

You can boost the benefits of this by breathing from the diaphragm.

Diaphragmatic breathing

Place one hand on your chest and the other over your belly button. As you breathe in, the hand on your stomach should be pushed out while the hand on your chest should not move. As you breathe out, your stomach should pull in. Your chest should not move.

To help, breathe in through your nose, purse your lips and breathe out slowly through your mouth. If you are a chest breather, you may find this difficult at first. If you can't get the hang of this, lie on your back on the floor and practise as it is easier to do in this position.

Put this together with the skills on the previous page. Once you get good at them, practise when you are at work, sitting on the bus, watching TV etc. The aim is to be able to do this no matter where you are if you feel you are beginning to hyperventilate. No one will notice what you are doing.

Controlling your thoughts

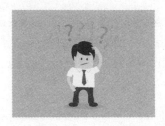

Think back to the vicious circle. It is the way you *interpret* the HV symptoms, not the HV itself, that causes the panicky feelings.

Combined with the breathing skills, getting a grip on your thoughts will really help. Again you should try to think your way out of feeling panicky. As in Chapter 6, first of all you have to:

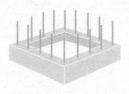

Build the foundation: stand back, pull back the blinkers, wait a minute.

Once you have built the foundation, it is time to **challenge**. Here are two of the Big 5 you could use:

What are the chances of . . . losing control or going mad?

> 'I always think I am going to lose control and crack up. I have felt like this lots of times in the past. But it doesn't happen. I don't go over the edge, even though I feel grim. These fears feed the panic feeling. If I can get a grip on them, I won't feel as panicky. And I now know I'm staying in my comfort zone too much. Get out of it and face the fear and fight it all the way.'

What is the worst thing that can happen . . . if I wake in a panic in the middle of the night?

> 'The worst thing that can happen is that I'll be full of fear. I'll feel that I can't breathe; I will end up in tears and feel awful. That is bad news, but it won't be the end of the world. And that is *if* it happens. I now have some weapons to use to fight it. I know that I can't come to harm so I can keep a lid on this fear.'

And, of course, **Breaking Stress Up** is perfect for those times when you know you are more likely to feel panicky. Preparing, facing up and reviewing allow you to prevent a big build-up and stay in control.

Work out your own ways to control your thoughts using these new skills.

Controlling your actions

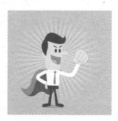

Look at what may happen to your **behaviour** and **avoidance**:

Behaviour
Do you:

Try to fill your lungs with air if you HV? Do you leave your bedroom window open to let more air in? You now know that you need *less* air, not more. So make sure your actions help not hinder you. So, if leaving your window open is an example of staying in your comfort zone, keep that window shut!

Pace up and down the room, try to read, watch TV – anything to try not to think about how you feel? Don't try to run from the panic feeling. Face it and fight back using the skills you have been learning.

Avoidance
Do you:

Avoid going to certain places because you think you will feel panicky there? *Go there, face it and do not run away.* Work out how to handle it and prepare well. Don't give in to it.

Avoid becoming emotional – feeling angry, feeling excited – in case it provokes a feeling of panic? Think of that skateboarding penguin. Allow all these normal emotions to come out. In the long run, the restrictions on your life are adding strength to the panic feeling. Don't give in to it.

Do things to try to stop feeling panicky – carry a diazepam, make sure there is someone at home with you? In the long run these actions make you worse, not better. Step out of your safety zone.

Whatever the action problems are, try hard to change the way you react to panic feelings. If you feel overwhelmed by the situations that trigger panicky feelings, use problem solving as a way to break up the problem into more manageable bits. By doing so you will show yourself that you can get a grip on this problem. Then your self-confidence and self-esteem will grow.

Reducing the risk of feeling panicky

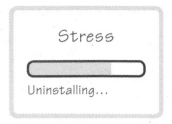

So far we have looked at ways of hitting panic feelings head on. Now let's look at some of the risk factors. Knowing what they are helps you plan ways to *prevent* panic feelings.

Rapid postural change

Don't change your position too fast. If you have been sitting down for a while, get out of the chair slowly. Don't jump out of bed first thing. You may get a swimming feeling in your head if you do. This can lead some people to feel panicky.

Tiredness

Make sure you get enough rest, as both panic feelings and stress are made worse by fatigue (and work hard at the skills you will learn to improve your sleep in Chapter 9).

Low (normal) blood sugar

This is nothing to do with diabetes. You keep your blood sugar level up when you eat. If you don't eat for a few hours the level drops and makes you more prone to feeling panicky. Though it slows down while you sleep, you need to eat something first thing to raise your sugar level – a piece of toast should be enough. Don't skip meals or go on crash diets. As a rough rule of thumb, eat something every three hours.

Alcohol

You may find you feel panicky 'the morning after the night before', even if you have not had a great deal to drink. If you are prone to this, stay away from drinking, at least in the short term. You can get into a vicious circle where you drink because you feel panicky and you feel panicky because you drink. This is the start of the slippery slope to big problems, so watch out for this. Drugs such as cocaine and speed can cause panicky feelings so for this – and many other reasons – you should steer clear of them.

Illness

Illnesses like the flu leave you more at risk. When you feel weak you are less able to fight off panic feelings. This may also be the case when you are recovering from illness.

Caffeine

Too much caffeine can be linked to panicky feelings. Caffeine can be found in coffee (much higher levels in fresh coffee), tea, fizzy drinks like Coke and Pepsi (including diet versions), pain-killers such as aspirin, some workout supplements, cold remedies and headache tablets. Chocolate contains caffeine, though at quite a low level. Many other products contain caffeine, so check the packets before using.

Effects of caffeine Feeling nervous, irritable, agitated, shaky, headaches, muscle twitch, flushed face, upset stomach, increased heart rate, speeded-up breathing, poor sleep (especially if you take caffeine at night). Your body can get so used to caffeine that, if you just cut it out dead, you can get:

Withdrawal effects Throbbing headache, tiredness or drowsiness, anxiety, depression and feeling sick. These feelings could last up to one week.

If you think caffeine may affect you, you should:

- Wean yourself off it slowly to avoid withdrawal effects.
- Switch to decaffeinated tea and coffee.
- Switch from fizzy drinks to caffeine-free drinks or pure fruit juice.
- Take as few painkillers, etc. as you can (check this with your GP if concerned).

See Chapter 5 for more information.

Premenstrual phase

Many women find that they are more prone to feeling panicky in the days before their period starts. This may be influenced by a natural drop in CO_2 levels at this stage in the cycle, and so HV kicks in more quickly. Of course, the symptoms of PMT may increase stress in any case. Women going through the menopause may also feel more prone to panicky feelings.

Stress

This is the most common risk factor. Control stress and you are well on the road to controlling panicky feelings. Knowing what your risk factors are can help you prevent panic attacks. Think of this scenario:

You have a late night with your friends. You are getting over a virus. Work is really stressful just now. You are premenstrual. You have a few drinks. You get back home at 4a.m. You get up early the next day, don't eat but have a few cups of strong coffee to get yourself going. This may not be your best day ever . . .

Plan ways to lower your risk In this case, cut down how much you drink, eat some toast first thing, take decaf coffee or fruit juice. You are at much less risk of feeling panicky now. Focus on what you can change, not on what you can't.

What to do if the panicky feeling grows into a panic attack

If you feel a panic attack come on, put this advice into action as quickly as you can. Nip the panic in the bud. It may help if someone can run through these steps with you. If you are alone, say them out loud.

- If you feel a panic attack coming on, stand your ground: don't let it make you run away. Step out of your comfort zone.
- Keep your breathing under control – slow, normal breaths. Each time you breathe in, say 'I'm in control'. Each time you breathe out, say 'Relax'.

- Relax your body – drop your shoulders, let your muscles go loose. Imagine the panic falling from the top of your head and down through your body, falling out of your toes.
- Keep your thoughts under control. Say 'I'm having a panic attack. I feel awful but nothing bad will happen. I know what to do. I can control this. It will pass.'

Fight the panic all the way. Rule it – don't let it rule you.

Last words

The aim of this chapter is to help you control and prevent panicky feelings. It takes time and hard work to get on top of this, so don't be put off by early problems. Keep at it. It will be well worth it in the end. Now look for ways to combine these skills with the ones you have learned in the previous chapters.

In Chapter 9 you will learn ways to control sleep problems. This will also help reduce panicky feelings (and much more).

9

Getting a good night's sleep

This chapter – the next step on the road to stress control – teaches you how to get a good night's sleep and so be better able to fight stress the next day.

Part 1 Information

Although there is much about sleep we don't yet know, we do know that getting a good night's sleep is vital for us. Here are four reasons why:

- It helps children to grow, both mentally and physically.
- It repairs our tired bodies.
- It sorts out our thoughts and memories.
- It boosts our well-being.

As we move towards the final stages of acquiring the necessary skills to beat stress, the vicious circle weakens further:

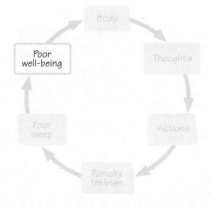

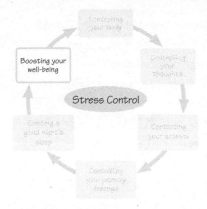

This chapter aims to teach skills that will help you get a good night's sleep and, as a result, lower your stress. At the same time, your confidence and self-esteem get a chance to grow. Recharging your batteries in this way helps to feed your positive circle:

The 'Sleep Cycle'

Sleep is made up of five stages. When we first fall asleep, we go into **Stage 1** sleep. This is a very light sleep. As you go into **Stage 2** and **Stage 3**, your sleep gets deeper. By **Stage 4**, you are in a very deep sleep.

You then go into a stage called Rapid Eye Movement (**REM**) sleep. This is when most of our dreams occur (we only recall our dreams if we wake up during this stage).

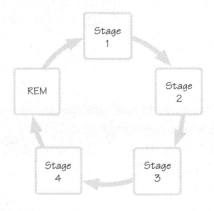

Once REM sleep is over, we go back to Stage 1 sleep. We may go through this cycle four or five times each night. It is normal to wake up at least once during the night. And as long as you get back to sleep quickly then it is nothing to worry about.

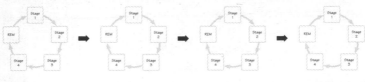

Night   Morning

We get more deep sleep at the start of the night; we get more REM sleep towards morning. Deep sleep helps our bodies recover; REM sleep helps our minds recover. So a lack of both can badly affect us during the day.

Common daytime signs of poor sleep are:

Dragging yourself through the day	Poor memory
Lethargy	Being irritable
Not 'on the ball'	Slower to react
Less vigilant	Hard to learn new things
Making daft mistakes	Poor concentration

A good night's sleep gets us in better shape to face the next day and in better shape to fight off stress.

Types of sleep problems

'It's weird:
I feel so tired when I get into bed,
but as soon as I put out the light I
start thinking about everything. And no matter
what I do, I can't get back to sleep. Yvonne
is fast asleep in seconds and I'm left
on my own, wide awake.'

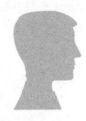

'I wake up
at two in the morning with a lot of
stupid thoughts going round and
round in my head. I just got up and I spend half
the night in the living room. I can't tell you how
lonely I feel then. And of course, during
the day, I am walking about half-asleep.'

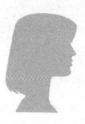

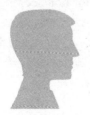

'I'm quite down just now
and I find that I'm awake at five in
the morning. I'll not get back to sleep
again, even though I want to. So I lie there
with all these dark thoughts. It is a bad
way to start the day.'

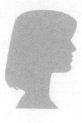

'I have to take a few drinks to get me to sleep. But I wake up within a few hours and that might be me for hours. I feel so miserable.'

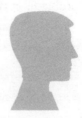

'I feel I sleep for a reasonable time but I never feel rested, that I've recharged my batteries. So I struggle to cope during the day as I feel as if I'm only half-awake. No energy, rubbish concentration. What I'd give for a solid night's sleep!'

Some reasons for poor sleep

Sleep problems can arise for a range of reasons. Here are some of the common ones:

Stress is, for many, the most important reason for not sleeping well. You may find, during the day, that you can cope OK as long as you keep busy and distracted. So, when you go to bed and switch off the light and have nothing to do, your mind switches on and goes into overdrive.

Shift work prevents you from getting into a good sleep habit. Too many night shifts are bad for both mind and body, but if you have no choice but to do shifts, work extra hard at the advice given under 'Getting a good night's sleep' (below).

Age As we get older we need less sleep, yet often we try to sleep for the same number of hours as we needed when we were younger.

Need to go to the toilet is often tied to age. As we get older, we are more likely to get up at least once each night. Illness can affect this need as well.

Pain and illness can affect our sleep. Physical problems such as arthritis can affect sleep quality. Sometimes the tablets we take to help combat illness might affect sleep. Your GP can check this for you.

Noise Often people living in noisy places sleep poorly. And no wonder if the neighbours are playing music till all hours or if your street is always busy. Maybe you can't do much about this; but you can reduce noise disturbance inside your own house.

Poor routine Think how important it is to get a toddler into a good bedtime routine. We're showing the child that the high energy of the day is at an end; that we're now slowing down to make it easier to drop off to sleep. As adults we often forget this and don't build in that 'calming down' period between the busy day and sleeping.

Caffeine speeds up the body and mind. It makes you much more alert (and possibly anxious) just at the time when you want to be shutting down. It can also cut back on deep sleep.

217

We will look at ways to overcome some of these problems later in the chapter.

Part 2 Getting a good night's sleep

Stage 1 Sleeping tips

- Your sleeping needs.
- Your bedroom.
- Calm your body.
- Calm your mind.
- Build up good habits.

Your sleeping needs

Age As we get older, we need less sleep (our bodies – and brains! – aren't growing much now). Once we get into middle age we get less deep sleep and so can be woken more easily. Most middle-aged people don't need as much sleep as they did when they were twenty. Are you perhaps trying to sleep too long for your needs? If so, try going to bed fifteen minutes later each week and see what amount of sleep works best for you.

Lifestyle The amount of sleep you need also depends on your lifestyle. So someone with a hectic lifestyle who expends a lot of energy each day will probably need more sleep than someone with a more sedate lifestyle.

This means having to balance age and lifestyle – a very active eighty-year-old may need more sleep than an eighteen-year-old couch potato.

Pills A quick word on sleeping tablets. Your GP will probably give you only a few (if any). This makes good sense as sleeping pills do not work in the long run (and often not at all). They change the type of sleep you get. Don't depend on them; there are much better ways to get a good night's sleep. Your GP may give you an antidepressant to use over a longer period. But, again, unless your doctor feels it could help low mood, it is better to learn the skills that can teach you to improve your sleep.

Your bedroom

Get the room fresh At some point in the day, open the windows to let in fresh air.

Get the room at the right temperature This is the 'Goldilocks Rule': the room should not be too hot or too cold. Around 64°F (18°C) is best. Too hot makes us more restless, gives us less REM sleep and tends to wake us up more. Too cold makes it harder to get to sleep and maybe leads to more nightmares.

Your bed If your bed is past its best, and if you can afford it, think about a new one. Make sure your pillows are right for you. Don't have a duvet that makes you too hot.

Light We are made to sleep in the dark. So make sure you have thick curtains or blackout blinds. An eyemask works fine. Try to avoid bright screens, e.g. on your tablet, while reading in bed. Due to the light it gives off, switch your phone off or leave it in another room during the night.

Noise If you can't stop the noise outside the house, use earplugs. You can also get an FM radio and tune it off the station so you get 'white noise'. This is good for swallowing up other disturbing noises. Use ear plugs.

Calm your body

Exercise Exercise can be helpful, but don't do this in the few hours before going to bed – early evening is perfect. A brisk thirty-minute walk is fine, or even two fifteen-minute walks. See Chapter 5 for more advice.

Food Avoid big meals in the few hours before bedtime. Your digestive system wakes up and starts to work hard just when you want your body to be calming down. A slice of toast or a biscuit before bed should be fine (bread and pasta can be good for making us drowsy). Avoid fatty or spicy food. Avoid red wine, cheese, nuts and bacon as these tend to wake us up.

Drink Try to reduce your liquid intake in the evening to reduce the likelihood of waking to go to the toilet.

Caffeine This wakes up our bodies. So cut back on tea, coffee, energy and fizzy drinks, some painkillers and headache tablets. Try to cut it out as much as you can from late afternoon onwards. See Chapter 5 for more advice.

Milky drinks The old wives were right! Ovaltine, Horlicks or hot milk might help you get to sleep. Take these instead of tea or coffee at bedtime.

Smoking Like caffeine, nicotine wakes up the body and keeps us alert. Try not to smoke for at least ninety minutes before bed. Never smoke if you wake up during the night. If you are a heavy smoker, you would be best to give up anyway. Ask your doctor for advice on ways of stopping.

Alcohol Never rely on alcohol to get to sleep. Although it can make you sleepy, it can also wake you up. It makes us snore more, affects our breathing and makes us more restless. It reduces deep sleep and REM sleep – the type of sleep we really want. It can add to our stress the next day. If you think alcohol is a problem, please see your GP for help.

Body temperature Apply the 'Goldilocks rule' (see above)! Don't have a hot bath or shower straight before bed. And try not to be too cold before jumping into bed.

Calm your mind
Worry time Set a time in the evening to do your worrying – say 8p.m. Do this well before your bedtime. So if you start to worry in the morning, stop yourself and 'save' the worry until your 'worry time'. Come 8p.m., stop what you are doing and worry about all the things you have stored up over the day. Chances are you will have forgotten them. Even if you do try to worry, you'll probably find it very hard to 'feel' the worry.

Arguments Try not to go to bed on an argument. So work hard to make up before you get into the bedroom.

Relaxation Use one of your relaxation techniques before going to, or when you are in, bed. Once you get good at it, you should be able to run the exercise through your head without having to listen to the audio track.

Build up good habits

Bedtime routine Do you have a bedtime routine? A transition between day and night? Give your body and mind a chance to build up a good routine. So go to bed at more or less the same time. Get up at the same time. Avoid long lie-ins. Build up a routine at night that slows you down and tells your body that you are getting ready for bed.

Relax before bed Think of ways to slow yourself down in the hour before going to bed. Decide what you want to do – read? listen to music? chat? watch TV? And do it. If you have just come in from a night out or off a back shift or if you are studying, make sure you give yourself a space in which to switch off and relax.

Tech detox See if you can avoid all technology in the hour before bed. Don't check emails, texts and/or social media while in bed.

Your partner If your partner snores or is restless, ask if he or she could move to another room. Your partner has to move – not you – as you have to learn to sleep well in your own bed. Once you are making progress, your partner can be invited back to sleep in the same bed.

Stage 2 Retraining your sleep

For those of you with long-standing sleep problems this is a great skill to acquire. It asks a lot of you but it will be well worth it in the end.

Note that you must follow the stages below to the letter.

The role of association

Maggie is a great sleeper. She falls asleep most nights within fifteen minutes. She may wake to go to the toilet but gets to sleep again in a few minutes. Her *associations* with bed are all good:

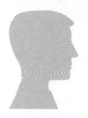

'This is the place where I get to sleep, where I feel safe, comfy, relaxed and content. I'll wake up refreshed and feeling that I've recharged my batteries.'

As Maggie slept well last night and the night before, she believes she will sleep well tonight. As she leaves the living room and walks towards her bedroom, everything is working in Maggie's favour. Her chances of sleeping well tonight are good.

On the other hand, we have poor Mark. He associates the bed with *not* sleeping.

'This is the place where I don't get to sleep; where I toss and turn, where I feel stressed, angry, frustrated. It's where I worry and feel down. It's where I wake up during the night and then can't get back to sleep again. This is a place where I never get a decent rest.'

As Mark didn't sleep well last night or the night before, he believes he is in for another bad night. As Mark leaves the living room and walks towards his bedroom, everything is working against him. His chances of sleeping well tonight are poor.

Retraining your sleep is all about changing your associations with your bed. There are six stages:

223

Stage 1 Don't go to bed until you feel sleepy

You no longer have a 'bedtime'. Only go to bed once you start to feel sleepy. Don't go to bed because the others are going to bed, because you feel bored or because it is bedtime. You must stay up until you feel tired *no matter how long this takes*.

Stage 2 Remember that your bedroom is only for sleeping

This step gets rid of the things that keep you from sleep. Reading a book in bed is fine if you don't have a sleep problem. But you need to *associate* the bed with sleeping *and nothing else*. If you are reading, you are not sleeping. So you should not read, watch TV, listen to the radio, check emails, phone friends, etc. Sex is OK, however, as it can help relax you and may help you get to sleep afterwards.

As soon as you get into bed, put the light out and try to sleep. Though you may know good sleepers who read in bed or watch TV, you must do these things outside the bedroom until you get on top of the problems.

Stage 3 If you don't fall asleep in twenty minutes, get up

If you are not asleep in twenty minutes, you may not be asleep in fifty. Think back to the idea of *association*. You don't want to associate bed with you tossing and turning, feeling stressed and so on. So after twenty minutes, go back to the living room. Don't watch TV. Don't eat or drink. You could read a magazine or listen to relaxing music. You must stay in the living room until you feel sleepy again *no matter how long this takes*. When you feel sleepy, go back to bed. At the start, you may be up a few times each night. It may be hard to get out of a warm bed, but you must do this.

Stage 4 Repeat (and repeat and repeat)

Repeat again and again if you have to. So you have twenty minutes in which to get to sleep each time you try. If you don't – it's back to the living room.

Stage 5 Get up early each morning

Get up no later than 8.30a.m. Set the alarm, and as soon as it goes off get up and out of the bedroom.

Even if you feel that you have hardly slept a wink, you must follow this to the letter. You should also try to do this seven days a week – no lie-ins at the weekend – until you get this problem sorted out.

Stage 6 Don't try to catch up on sleep

You may want to nap during the day to catch up on lost sleep, e.g. after a meal. Don't do it. Save the sleep for bedtime.

Work out when you most want to sleep during the day. Then work out a way of making sure that you don't fall into the trap: go out for a walk, phone a friend, etc.

Keep at it

This is a great skill but it is also a hard one to stick to. It makes great demands on you in the first few nights. It is very tempting to stay in bed after twenty minutes, to have a long lie-in or afternoon nap because you can hardly keep your eyes open. Fight these urges the whole way.

Don't expect rapid change. Your poor sleep may have built up over a long time, so it will take time to get better. It will be well worth it in the long run.

Keeping a practice form can be a good way to plot your progress.

Sleep practice form

Each morning, keep a note of the following:

Rate the quality of your sleep between 1 and 10, where 10 = perfect night's sleep.

What time did you try to go to sleep?
How long did it take you to fall asleep?
How often did you wake during the night?
How long did it take you to fall asleep each time?
When did you wake?
When did you get up?

Last words

The aim of Chapter 9 is to help you get a good night's sleep, and so recharge your batteries. This can have a huge effect on daytime stress. The better you sleep, the easier it will be to control your stress. And, of course, the more you control your stress, the easier it will be to get a good night's sleep.

In the next chapter you will learn some great ways to boost your well-being. These skills will help you weaken the vicious circle and further strengthen the positive circle.

10

Well-being

This book has taught you a lot about stress, and a lot about how to fight it. To help you stay in control (and to help you even more) this chapter looks at boosting well-being and resilience using positive psychology and mindfulness skills.

Part 1 Information

And so, at last, we shut off the fuel supply feeding the vicious circle.

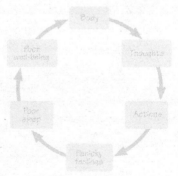

As we reach a state of well-being, the positive circle is complete. All the skills we have learned so far come together and help produce stress control.

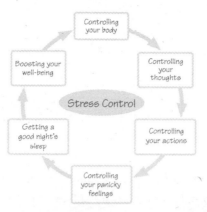

So far, we have focused on getting control over *bad* emotions – anxiety, depression, panic, etc. Now we are ready to look at boosting *good* emotions: happiness, gratitude, compassion, etc. Once we combine these two strands, we will have a set of skills that will help keep us in control and more able to cope with what life throws at us. But good well-being is more than just having control over stress. It is also about feeling comfortable, contented and healthy. Or, if life is against you just now and it would be unreasonable to expect to feel content or happy, well-being can give you the resilience to cope with the bad times.

In the past it was felt that controlling stress would, in itself, lead to well-being. We now know there is more to it than that. To make sense of this we need to understand the 'stress line':

Low stress   High stress

Everyone in the world is somewhere on this line (and, of course, our place on the line can change hour by hour, minute by minute). Now we have to add a well-being line:

229

Good well-being

Poor well-being

Just as with the stress line, everyone can be placed somewhere on this line, and we know that our position can change in an instant. We often call good well-being 'flourishing' and poor well-being 'languishing'. Now we have to combine the lines, giving us four boxes:

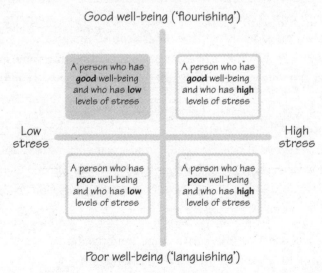

Of course, people can move from box to box, but you may be able to work out in which box you would place yourself. Go back to Chapter 3 and check your score on the stress measures – the PHQ-9 and the GAD-7 – and the well-being measure – the WEMWBS – to give you an idea where you would place yourself. You can see that it is possible to have good well-being even in the face of high stress, or to have poor well-being in the face of low stress. But what we want to achieve is the best of both worlds: good well-being and low stress – the highlighted box.

We can divide well-being into three areas:

Languishing 'Languishers' often describe their lives as 'hollow' or 'empty'. They feel their lives lack meaning and purpose; that they can do little to change their lives as they lack control. They may feel unhappy, unfulfilled and isolated. They are prone to poor health and very prone to stress.

Middling This is where most of us are – somewhere in between.

Flourishing The opposite of languishing. 'Flourishers' feel good about their lives – optimistic, happy, in control. They feel they have the power to make changes in their lives. Their health benefits and it protects them against stress. It even helps them live longer.

Once we learn how to control stress we have built a strong foundation, putting us in a good position to boost well-being and enabling us to 'flourish'. Better well-being then protects us against stress becoming a problem in the future. It is another positive circle.

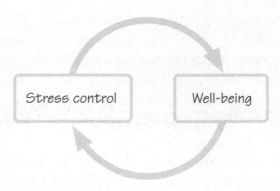

Flourishing

When our well-being is high and we flourish, we are more likely to feel:

- Respected by those around us (and more able to respect them);
- Close to others;
- That we 'belong';
- Valued;
- More in control of our lives;
- More creative;
- Able to make changes in our lives;
- Able to take advantage of opportunities;
- More able to cope with adversity.

While this helps us feel good, it does a *lot* more:

- Improves our health;
- Helps keep our stress at a low level;
- Helps prevent future problems with stress;

- Reduces the likelihood of smoking;
- Reduces the likelihood of drinking too much, especially binge-drinking;
- Reduces visits to the doctor;
- Reduces medication;
- Reduces the likelihood of going to hospital;
- Reduces blood pressure;
- Protects us from heart attacks, strokes and other serious health problems;
- Reduces the risk of chronic physical illness;
- Helps us live longer (around an extra seven years).

Neighbourhood and workplace issues

In general, as deprivation increases, well-being (like stress) gets worse. Countries with very unequal societies have, on the whole, poorer well-being. Other 'life' issues that make it more likely that people 'languish' are:

- Living in an 'unfair' society;
- A sense of being excluded and isolated;
- Loneliness;
- Unemployment;
- Low income;
- Poor housing;
- Debt and financial insecurity;
- The threat of violence;
- Bad life events: relationship breakdown, illness and bereavement, etc.

These are all bad things and, sadly, many are out of our control. But the good news is that there are things we can do to protect ourselves. This chapter will look at how each of us can become more resilient.

But we also need to look at the bigger picture.

At a wider level, solid neighbourhoods can make a big difference, even in very poor areas. So communities can also 'flourish', and this is more likely where:

- Neighbourhoods are strong – where people feel they 'belong';
- In neighbourhoods where people feel more secure;
- A lot of local people play a role in keeping their community together;
- There are good transport links;
- There are good local leisure facilities;
- There is the chance to learn new skills.

Workplaces also have a big role to play in well-being: ensuring a safe and secure working environment, decent working conditions, fair pay, job security, good work-life balance, achievable workload, good management, no culture of bullying, sense of control, etc. Creating conditions like this allows the workplace to 'flourish'.

This then helps each of us flourish, and our resilience builds. That feeds back into both the neighbourhood and the workplace, helping them flourish more. It's a win-win situation. And so another positive circle is built. So while this chapter looks at making each of us more resilient, think about wider change – think about how you can also help your community and workplace grow. If enough of us do this, our whole country could 'flourish'. And that's an ambitious goal: statistics show that around 3 in 10 of us 'languish', 5 out of 10 are in the middle and only 2 in 10 of us 'flourish'. The big task in the twenty-first century is to move as many of us as possible towards 'flourishing'. This book, I hope, will play a part in achieving this goal.

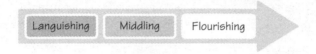

Boosting your well-being skills

Part 1 Four steps to well-being

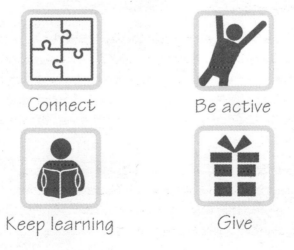

Part 2 Mindfulness

Take notice

Part 3 Be the best version of you

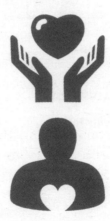

Part 1 Four steps to well-being

I am indebted to the New Economics Foundation (NEF) who developed these ideas.

Connect

. . . with the people around you. Your family, friends, neighbours, workmates. Work hard to make and then keep these relationships strong.

'Belonging' is crucial to well-being. Having solid relationships helps us to flourish by boosting our self-esteem and self-confidence. We all benefit but (and this may be a surprise to many) the people who most benefit from having a strong, close relationship are men. And what seems to be important here is that they *know*, in their heart of hearts, that that special person will be there for them if times get bad.

Getting support from others helps us over the hard times. Giving support helps us feel that we are decent, worthwhile people. Feeling connected gives us a sense that we are part of something bigger, and this helps boost well-being.

So think about your relationships: are they strong? Is there someone there for you? Are there people who know they can rely on you? Are you involved enough in the wider world? If so, great – keep working hard to maintain this. If you feel you need to boost your relationships, ask yourself what you need to do: are you sidelining them due to spending too much time on work? Is shyness holding you back? Do you have too many commitments elsewhere in your life? Do you need to get a better balance in life?

Think about:

- Making time each day to be with people.
- Organizing a day out or a trip into town for a drink, etc.
- Switching off the TV tonight, phoning a friend, playing a game with the children, or just talking.
- Finding out what is happening in your community and getting involved.
- Helping out a friend or family member who could do with some support.

Be active

Go for a walk or a run. Head outside. Cycle. Tend the garden. Dance. Exercise makes you feel good. Find something you enjoy doing. A brisk thirty-minute walk each day can work wonders for you.

Healthy body, healthy mind. In Chapter 5 we looked at the link between exercise and stress. Hopefully you are now trying to get thirty minutes' exercise most days of the week. Make sure this is something you enjoy so that you will be more likely to keep it going.

However, we also looked at the other benefits being active can bring: a sense of purpose and new goals – these also help us to 'flourish'. So this is more than just exercise; it is about actively engaging with life. So think about being active in a wider sense: get up at a reasonable hour even if you are not working, get dressed and 'get going' instead of lounging about (there's nothing wrong with doing this now and then, but don't get into the habit).

And think about tying this in with other well-being ideas. If you join a yoga class, a choir or a volunteer group, you start to *connect to* new people. As you feel the benefits of connecting you are more likely to stay e.g. at the class and your well-being rises further.

Keep learning

Try something new. Pick up an old interest. Sign up for a course. Take on a new responsibility at work. Fix something. Learn to cook something new. Give yourself a challenge. Learning new things builds confidence. And it can be good fun.

Learning new things is a great way to keep your brain ticking over. And the great thing about this is that a very wide range of learning works – you don't need to sign up for a college course or study for an exam (although that's fine if that's what you want to do) – you can learn a new sport, a new recipe, read a book, spend an hour on Wikipedia, learn a new skill from YouTube, fix something in the house.

Just as with 'be active', this can give us a sense of purpose via new goals and challenges. There is little better than the feeling of achievement when we master a new skill.

And think about tying this into other well-being ideas. So, if you join a night class or join an online forum, you start to *connect* to new people. If you learn a new sport, you are *more active*. As you feel the benefits of connecting and being active, it helps you keep your learning going.

Give

Do something nice for a friend or a stranger. Thank someone. Smile. Volunteer your time. Join a community group. Look out, as well as in. Seeing yourself, and your happiness, linked to the wider community, can be very rewarding and helps build connections with the people around you.

The big message here is that giving to others helps us too. And it can be a very simple act – chatting to a lonely neighbour, helping out at the church fête, offering to swop a shift with a workmate – that makes us feel we are better people. Amazingly, it can also alter our brains, helping us feel better about ourselves.

The constant flood of advertising claims try to make us believe that we can only be happy if we have the latest TV, trainers, phone, etc. But as we all really know, we need to search for well-being elsewhere, and 'giving' is a great place to start.

So offer a hand whenever you can, whether this is to help a workmate or a friend who needs a bit of help. You could think of volunteering to help those in your community who are struggling. Looking after one another will help strengthen our villages, towns and cities.

And think about tying this in with other well-being ideas. If you give your time to others, you are connecting with them; instead of sitting in front of the TV you are more active, and the chances are you will be learning something new at the same time. Combining this with the sense of purpose and 'doing the right thing' will help us feel better about ourselves and so move towards 'flourishing'.

Part 2 Mindfulness

Be curious. Notice the world around you – the views, the sounds, the smells. Notice the changing seasons. Savour the moment whether you are on the bus, eating a meal or talking to friends. Be aware of what you are feeling. Reflect on your experiences.

Many of us spend too much time on autopilot, moving through life without stopping to notice the things that are going on around us. We can do housework, sit on a bus, eat a meal, drive a car, walk down the road and yet be miles away in our minds. This isn't always a bad thing – it can be enjoyable thinking about happy times, things we are going to do, daydreaming, using our imagination and so on.

However, when we are stressed our minds tend to get into bad habits. These autopilot moments act like magnets that attract bad thoughts and feelings: worry, brooding, being upset and so on. We are back to the blinkers of controlling your thoughts. We are trapped in the 'what ifs' of the future and the 'if onlys' of the past while, on the wrong side of the blinkers, the present passes us by. It is all too easy to lose touch with ourselves. This section looks at mindfulness as a way to pull back the blinkers to allow us to get back in touch. By so doing, we then further boost our well-being.

Mindfulness helps us to:

- Live in the moment.
- Shift the focus of our attention away from *thinking* about our worries and concerns to *observing* our feelings, thoughts or body with curiosity and in detail.
- Practise acceptance, i.e. paying attention to our feelings and thoughts but not judging them – just letting them exist without trying to sort them out.
- Get back in touch with ourselves.

Learning to become mindful makes us more aware when bad thoughts are getting on top of us but also able to accept that these thoughts do not have to control us.

So the perfect strapline for this is:

Take notice

... our thoughts, feelings and body sensations and what is going on around us moment by moment.

If you want to sum this up in one phrase, it is this: **stop and smell the roses.**

In mindfulness, you don't let yourself get *tangled up* in these thoughts but, instead, detach from them, *observe* them and let them go. Doing mindful exercises stops us being on automatic pilot. This gives us a greater sense of well-being and control as all the worries and distress don't get pulled into our mind as easily. The next section gives you some great ways to become mindful.

Mindful skills

Give the grasshopper a rest.

In Chapter 6 we looked at how grasshopper thinking led stress to build up quickly. Now that you have learned the controlling your thoughts skills like building the foundation (stand back, pull back the blinkers, wait a minute), we can use mindfulness to pay attention to the present. Try these skills to 'calm the grasshopper' by stopping him jumping from one thought to the next.

Everyday mindfulness

To start the mindful process, simply become more aware of everyday activities. Be mindful of eating your meal: look in detail at the food on the plate, feel it in your mouth, experience the taste, the smell. Be aware of it as you chew. This is not about seeking out beauty; you can be mindful of anything in your world. What you are doing is noticing your world in a new way.

So next time you are outside, be mindful – be mindful of your walking as your feet hit the ground. What can you hear? What can you see? What can you smell? Can you feel the wind on your face? What are the thoughts in your mind (just observe and accept them)? The sounds, sights and so on do not need to be pleasant. Just be mindful of them – this is your world. Take time to smell the roses.

Mindful breathing

This is a simple but useful exercise. Just focus on your breathing for one minute. You can do this anywhere, anytime, whether sitting or standing. Think back to Chapter 4 and the skill of 'calm breathing': breathe in slowly through your nose for a count of three to four seconds. Hold this for three to four seconds and breathe out through your mouth over a count of six to eight seconds. Repeat this three times.

Now add mindfulness to this skill. So really focus on each breath, and nothing else. If your mind does wander, don't worry – simply be aware of the thoughts. Let them be what they are. Don't try to change them but gently shift your focus back to your breathing. Be aware of taking in each breath through your nose; be aware of how it feels to hold each breath; how it feels as you breathe out through your mouth. Notice any changes to any other part of your body while doing this.

Mindful reflection

Find something in your world you can focus on. If outside it could be a tree, a cloud, the moon, a flower, a car; indoors it could simply be a clock, pen, chair or laptop. Anything. Focus just on it. As before, if thoughts come into your mind, let them be and let them disappear as you refocus on the object. Focus on it as if you are seeing it for the very first time. Explore the way it looks, maybe the way it feels, the way it changes. Do this for a minute or two.

Leaves in the stream

Begin with mindful breathing. Close your eyes and become aware of the thoughts in your mind and, as you notice each thought, imagine placing it on a leaf and seeing that leaf float down the stream. Place every thought you notice on a leaf and watch it float away. Just let the thoughts come. If your attention wanders, gently bring your focus back to the thought and place it on the leaf.

After a minute or so, focus again on your mindful breathing, open your eyes, and become aware of your surroundings.

The body scan

This is a form of meditation that you can do every day, or however often that feels right for you. It helps put you more in touch with your body and helps you identify how you feel. As with the progressive relaxation and belly breathing from Chapter 5, it aims to help release any stress in your body.

Decide what ideas and exercises suit you best and practise as often as you can so that being mindful becomes second nature to you.

Audio clips to guide you through the body scan and leaves in the stream exercises, as well as the other relaxation tracks, can be found at www.stresscontrolaudio.com. Written instructions for both can be found in the Appendix.

Part 3 Be the best version of you

Learning and practising the skills of connect, be active, keep learning, give and take notice form the bedrock of well-being. Now, to boost their power, we can add **compassion** and **gratitude**.

Compassion

'If you want others to be happy, practise compassion. If you want to be happy, practise compassion.' The Dalai Lama

Stress often brings out the worst in us – we are moody, irritable, quick to anger, small-minded, etc. We can be hard to live with. So just when we want to 'connect' to boost our well-being, others may not be so keen to connect to us. But, as the vast majority of us are decent people trying our best in life, we try hard to act decently to others. So we try to have good relationships with others. Sadly, what we tend to do is save the real venom for ourselves. We talk to ourselves in ways we would never talk to any other human being; we put ourselves down, we never give ourselves credit, we even hate ourselves. So, as a result, the one relationship we really need to sort out is often not with others, it is with ourselves.

Time to think of those blinkers again. What is on the wrong side of the blinkers is our sense of compassion, even our sense of fairness – if you wouldn't talk to anyone else like this, why is it fair to talk to yourself in this way? You can't feel good about yourself if you keep this up. So you need to add to well-being by treating yourself with more compassion. This takes time and effort. It is easy, when you are stressed, to think of all the bad things – they are right in the middle of the blinkers. It's harder to see the good things about yourself.

So, as before, you must build the foundation – stand back, pull back the blinkers, wait a minute. And, with the blinkers back, give yourself a chance to see a more compassionate view of things. Then you can challenge the venom you use to talk to yourself. Also look back to the 'strengths' section in your life inventory (Chapter 3). Do these help?

To make this easier, here are two good ways to allow yourself to feel compassion:

The compassionate letter Before starting this task, carry out the mindful breathing we looked at earlier in the chapter and keep it going as you work through the process.

Imagine what your compassionate self is like – what would he/she think of the things that you give yourself a hard time over? As this person – the best version of you – write your usual self a letter. As the compassionate you, consider if you feel your usual self is being too critical; whether your usual self is missing out anything (make sure you have pulled back the blinkers); whether your usual self deserves more of a break.

Bear in mind that you are using the same skills you learned in controlling your thoughts where you had your common sense voice challenge your stress voice.

You might show this letter to someone who knows you well and whom you can trust. They might have some useful advice.

Compassionate actions This adds to the ideas covered in the four steps to well-being – think of 'connect' and 'give'. Simply put, the more you can care for others, the more you will be able to care for yourself. Helping can give meaning to our lives. We connect with others and realize that we all have our problems to cope with. And that helping one another on the journey through life benefits us all. Small acts of kindness can go a long way. So work hard to show compassion to friends, neighbours, workmates, family.

This is about becoming the kind of person you want to be (and surely all of us would like to be compassionate).

Finally, make sure that when you wake up each day you tell yourself to show compassion to yourself. A good idea is to carry a small stone on your pocket and, when you feel it, remember the importance of compassion and the small acts of kindness. And you can build on this by learning more about gratitude.

Gratitude

There is now a lot of evidence to show that feeling grateful can produce major changes in our lives: it makes us more generous, more helpful and compassionate. It reduces our sense of isolation and makes us more outgoing and forgiving. It can make us feel more alert and alive. It gives us a greater sense of pleasure in the everyday. Amazingly, it can change our brains, boost our immune systems, help us deal with aches and pains better and can lower blood pressure and heart rate.

Feeling grateful helps us to stay in the present rather than brood about the past or worry about the future (note the link to mindfulness). It helps block bad emotions like stress, envy and resentment. If you are more able to count your blessings you are, surely, less able to focus on the bad things. Grateful people are healthier, more satisfied and fulfilled. Simply saying 'Thank you' (and meaning it) can make us feel happier.

While some of us find it easy to be grateful for what we have got, many struggle – advertisers are constantly telling us that what we have isn't enough; that there is always something better we can buy; something better over the horizon. And although, sadly, there are many people in our society who do not have enough, many of us know that buying more doesn't lead to well-being.

So gaining a stronger sense of gratitude takes time and effort. Here are some great ways to achieve it and to become the best version of you:

Find three good things in your day At the end of the day, sit back and think about things you can be grateful for: your family, your job, your health. It could be a small act of kindness by a workmate. It could be a pleasant walk, a chat with a neighbour, a sunset. Some people keep a gratitude diary so they can go through it from time to time to remind themselves of the good things in their life. Do this as often as you want – once a day, once a week, once a month. Make sure it stays fresh, rather than just going over the same things each time.

Thank those to whom you feel grateful This can help them feel valued (they may not realize how you feel). Plus, if they feel valued, they are more likely to keep acting in a kind way to other people.

Gratitude letter Think of the people you feel gratitude towards but have been unable to tell. Sitting down and writing to them can be a very positive action. You may want the person to receive the letter or email, or you may not. You do not have to actually send it; just writing it may be enough for you to benefit (although think how wonderful that person would feel to receive your letter). The letter could be written to someone no longer alive – a grandparent, your first teacher, the person who ran your football team – but if you realize that person helped you along the way, consider what you want to say to them and sit down and write the letter.

Final words

Boosting well-being and controlling stress give you the greatest chance of long-term benefits. Think about the skills that suit you best and practise them from today, every day.

The final part of the jigsaw is covered in Chapter 11.

11

Controlling your future

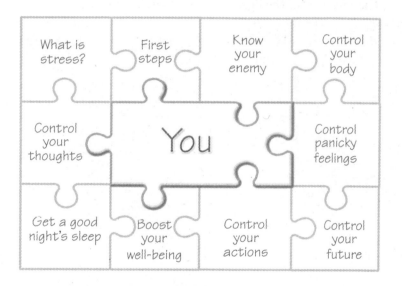

In this final chapter we will look at the best ways of combining the skills we have learned together to keep you on top of your life.

At the start of this book we looked at how stress keeps replenishing itself via a vicious circle, leaving you feeling overwhelmed:

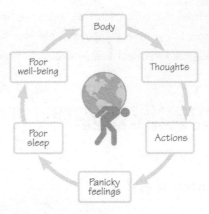

We end with a new positive circle in its place to achieve stress control and flourishing well-being:

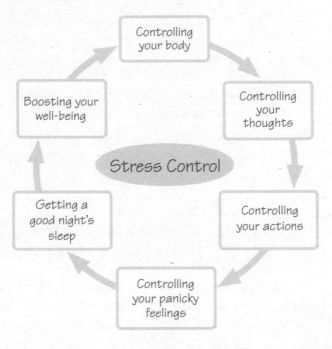

And now we must make sure that we keep feeding this positive circle to guarantee a better future. This can be achieved by using the skills we have learned in the five steps contained in this book.

Five steps to a better future

Step 1 Know your enemy

Chapter 2 What is stress?

You should now know a lot more about stress.

Chapter 3 Know your enemy

You should have described your stress and worked out the patterns.

- You should have completed the life inventory.
- You should have measured your stress and well-being.
- You should have drawn your vicious circle.
- You should have set your goals.

Step 2 First steps

Chapter 4

- You should have cleared the decks.
- You should have looked for hidden problems.
- You should have used some of the twenty-five ways of coping.

Step 3 Fighting back

Chapter 5 Controlling your body

- You should have looked at reducing caffeine.
- You should have looked at using exercise.
- You should have tried breathing retraining.
- You should have tried progressive relaxation.

Chapter 6 Controlling your thoughts

- You should know how to build the foundation.
- You should know how to use the Big 5 Challenges.
- You should know how to break stress up.

Chapter 7 Controlling your actions

- You should be facing your fear.
- You should have looked at stepping out of your comfort zone.
- You should have tried problem solving.

Chapter 8 Controlling your panicky feelings

- You should be combining your skills: controlling your body, thoughts and actions.
- You should have looked at reducing the risk of panic.

Chapter 9 Getting a good night's sleep

- You should have looked at the sleeping tips.
- You should have looked at retraining your sleep.

Step 4 Well-being

Chapter 10 Well-being

- You should have measured your well-being.
- You should have taken your four steps to well-being: connect, be active, keep learning, give.
- You should have studied everyday mindfulness; mindful breathing; mindful observation; leaves in the stream and the body scan.
- You should have practised being the best version of you with compassion and gratitude.

Step 5 Staying on top of your stress

Now that you have learned so much about stress and well-being, the hard work can begin. It is like passing your driving test: you know what to do, but you have to practise hard before you become a good driver. Choose the skills that seem most suited to you and work hard at them.

Goals for the future

When our stress is high it can sometimes seem simpler to take things one day at a time. And that can be a useful tactic. However, now that you are working on your future goals, you can start to think of the kind of future you want. Having goals motivates and challenges us and, if we reach our goal, a sense of accomplishment. They boost our self-confidence and self-belief. So think of what your goals could be. They should be *your* goals, and not those suggested by other people. The best way to do this is to use SMART criteria when setting your goals:

Specific Work out exactly what you want to achieve. Why will this be good for you? Can it be broken down into smaller steps? (Use problem solving here.)

Measurable How will you know when you reach your goal (or each step on the way)? Make your goals as clear-cut as you can.

Achievable Challenge yourself but make sure the goal is within your grasp. Do you have enough control to achieve your goal?

Relevant Useful questions might be: 'Is this a worthwhile goal?' 'Is this the best time to go for it?'

Time-bound This gives you a time-frame: 'When can I start it?' 'Where will I be in one month's time?' 'When will I reach my goal?'

Think carefully about your goals and write them down using SMART criteria.

Controlling your future

Take charge of your life

Aim for *active* not *passive* coping. Passive coping is, for example, when you hope someone else deals with a problem or that it will just go away. Active coping is when you take control, find out what the problem is and take responsibility for tackling it (problem solving is perfect for this).

Dealing with setbacks

Don't expect progress to be easy or smooth. Setbacks are common. Aim to slowly increase the number of good days and decrease the number of bad days.

Try to predict when a setback is more likely – if there are problems in the house, stress at work, after drinking too much, etc. Work out ways to prevent it.

Don't panic if you have a setback. Accept what is going on. Stand back and work out why it's happening. Then work out what you can do about it.

Don't see a setback as putting you back at square one. If you have taken five steps forward and something puts you back one step, you are still four steps up on the deal.

Let others help you

Express your feelings to them and get things off your chest. Choose people you can trust to help you. Be comforted by their concern. Listen to their advice. If the advice is sound, act on it.

Learn to pat yourself on the back

If you have reached any of the goals you have set; if you faced and then solved a problem; if you fought back worry, then you deserve praise – give yourself some straight away.

Build up supports

Stress can build up when you lack a range of supports in your life. If you have problems in one area you can lean on other supports until you sort out the problem. The moral is: don't put all your eggs in one basket.

Make sure you keep relationships strong. Build up new interests, new hobbies. Work on your social life. Make sure you have a structure to your day or week. Focus on the well-being ideas in the previous chapter.

Watch out for the slippery slope

Watch that old bad habits don't creep into your life. These could be to do with avoiding, cutting yourself off from others, drinking to control stress, allowing the grasshopper to leap without challenge. Jump in and stop these dead.

Look into the future

Don't leave things to chance – think and plan ahead. To make your progress easier, think about the following:

- What have been the most important things I have learned from reading this book?
- What have been the most (and least) useful skills I have learned?
- When are setbacks most likely and how can I prevent them?

- What aspects of stress am I not getting to grips with? Why is this and how can I best deal with this?

Last words

Each of the chapters in this book has been one piece of the jigsaw which, once put together, has allowed us to see the bigger picture that leads to stress control. The major theme running all the way through has been the aim of turning you into your own therapist. So now the final, and most important, piece of the jigsaw can be slotted into place – you.

Believe in yourself

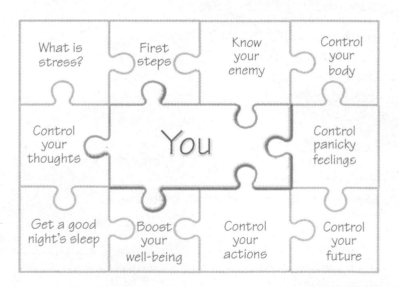

What is stress?   First steps   Know your enemy   Control your body

Control your thoughts   You   Control panicky feelings

Get a good night's sleep   Boost your well-being   Control your actions   Control your future

Because *you* matter.

Appendix 1

Relaxation and mindfulness

now https: stresscontrol.org

* Audio tracks available at www.stresscontrolaudio.com

Progressive relaxation 1: Deep relaxation

Settle back, as comfortably as you can. Let yourself relax to the best of your ability. Now clench your right fist, tighter and tighter, and study the tension as you do so. Keep it clenched and feel the tension in your right fist, hand and forearm . . . and now relax. Let the fingers of your right hand become loose. Observe the contrast in your feelings.

Now let yourself go and try to become relaxed all over. And once more, clench your right fist really tight. Hold it and notice the tension again . . . and let go, relax. Your fingers straighten out and you notice the difference once more.

Now repeat the process with your left fist. Clench your left fist while the rest of your body relaxes. Clench that fist tighter and feel the tension . . . relax . . . and feel the difference. Continue relaxing like that for a while and, as you do so, allow your breathing to slow down and let it become rhythmic and relaxed. And now clench both fists tighter and tighter; both fists tense,

263

forearms tense. Study the sensations, feel the tension . . . and relax. Straighten out your fingers and feel that relaxation. Continue relaxing your hands and forearms more and more.

Now bend your elbows and tense your upper arms; tense them harder and study the tension feelings . . . and now straighten out your arms, let them relax and feel that difference again. And let the relaxation develop and once more, tense your upper arms. Hold the tension and observe it carefully. Now straighten the arms and . . . relax. Relax as well as you can. And pay close attention to your feelings each time you tense and each time you relax.

Now straighten your arms so that you feel most tension along the back of your arms. Stretch your arms and feel that tension . . . and now relax. Get your arms back into a comfortable position and let the relaxation proceed on its own. Your arms should feel comfortably heavy as you allow them to relax. And, once more, straighten the arms so that you can feel the tension along the back of your arms. Straighten them, feel the tension, hold the tension . . . and relax. Just concentrate on pure relaxation in your arms and get rid of any tension. Get your arms comfortable and let them relax further and further . . . and continue relaxing your arms further and further. Even when your arms feel fully relaxed, try to go that extra bit further. Try to achieve deeper and deeper levels of relaxation.

Concentrate on relaxing your breathing. Slow down your breathing so it becomes nice and relaxed, rhythmic and relaxed. Just slow down your breathing and allow yourself to become more and more relaxed.

And let all your muscles go loose and heavy. Just settle back quietly and comfortably. Wrinkle up your forehead now, wrinkle it up tighter and tighter ... and now stop wrinkling your forehead. Relax and smooth it out. Picture your forehead and scalp becoming smoother as the relaxation increases. And now frown, crease your brows and study the tension. Hold the tension ... and then let it go. Smooth out the forehead once more.

And now close your eyes, tighter and tighter; feel the tension around the eyes. Hold the tension ... then let the tension go, and relax. Keep your eyes closed gently and comfortably and notice the relaxation and enjoy the relaxation. Now clench your jaws; bite your teeth together. Study the tension throughout the jaws. Hold the tension, feel the tension throughout the jaws ... and let the tension go. Let your lips part slightly and enjoy the relaxation. Now press your tongue hard against the roof of your mouth. Look for the tension ... and let the tension go. Let your tongue return to a relaxed and comfortable position. Now purse your lips together, tighter and tighter. Purse your lips and feel that tension ... and let the tension go. And note the contrast between tension and relaxation. Feel the relaxation all over your face, over your forehead and scalp. Eyes, jaws, lips, tongue and throat. The relaxation progresses further and further.

Now attend to your neck muscles. Press your head back as far as it can go and feel the tension in your neck. Roll it to the right and feel the tension shift. Roll it to the left; straighten your head and bring it forward; press your chin against your chest and let your head return to a comfortable position . . . and study the relaxation. Just let the relaxation develop.

Now shrug your shoulders; push them up as high as they will go. Push up your shoulders; hold the tension . . . and drop your shoulders and feel the relaxation. Your neck and shoulders relax. And, once again, push your shoulders up; push them up as high as they will go. Push them up, and forward, and back. Feel the tension in your shoulders and upper back. And then drop your shoulders once more and relax. Let the relaxation spread deep into the shoulders, right into your back muscles. Relax your neck and throat and your jaw and let your face become more and more relaxed. And let the relaxation grow deeper and deeper and deeper.

And again concentrate on slowing down your breathing. Let your breathing slow down so it too helps your body to relax more and more. Try to relax your whole body to the best of your ability. Feel that comfortable heaviness that goes along with relaxation and breathe easily and freely, in and out. Notice how the relaxation increases when you breathe out. Now breathe in deeply and fill your lungs. Hold your breath and study the tension . . . and now breathe out. Let the walls of your chest go loose and push the air out automatically. Continue relaxing and breathe freely and gently and slowly. Just feel the relaxation and enjoy it and, with the rest of your body as relaxed as possible, fill your lungs again. Breathe in deeply and hold it again. Breathe out and appreciate the difference. Continue to relax your chest and let the feelings spread to your back, shoulders, neck and arms. Just let go and enjoy the relaxation.

Now let's pay attention to your abdominal muscles. Tighten your stomach muscles. Make your abdomen hard. Notice the tension, hold the tension . . . and relax. Let the muscles loosen and notice the contrast. Once more, tighten your stomach muscles. Hold the tension and study it. Hold the tension and be aware of the tension . . . and let it go. Allow your stomach to relax more and more. Now draw your stomach in; pull the muscles in and feel the tension this way . . . and relax. Just let your stomach out; continue breathing normally and easily and feel the gentle massaging action all over your chest and stomach. Now pull your stomach in again and hold the tension. Now push out and feel the tension like that. Hold the tension. Once again, pull in and hold the tension . . . and now relax. Allow your stomach to relax fully. Let the tension dissolve as the relaxation grows deeper. And each time you breathe out, notice the rhythmic relaxation both in your lungs and in your stomach. Notice how your chest and your stomach relax more and more. And allow these feelings to develop right through your whole body as you become more and more relaxed. Let go of all tension and just relax.

Now flex your buttocks and thighs; flex by pushing down your heels as hard as you can. Really push them down . . . and relax . . . and notice the difference. Straighten your knees and flex your thigh muscles again. Hold the tension . . . and let it go. Let the relaxation proceed on its own.

Press your feet and toes downwards so that your calf muscles become tense. Study that tension; hold that tension . . . and let it go. This time, bend your feet up towards your face so that you can feel tension along your shins. Bring your toes right up; feel that tension . . . and let it go. Keep relaxing for a while.

Now let yourself relax further and further. Relax your feet, ankles, calves and shins. Relax your knees, thighs, buttocks and hips. Feel the heaviness of your lower body as you relax still further. And now let the relaxation spread to your stomach, waist and lower back. Let go more and more. Feel that relaxation all over. Let your upper back, chest, shoulders and arms, right to the tips of your fingers, relax more and more. Keep relaxing more and more deeply. Don't let any tension creep into your throat. Relax your neck and your jaw and all the muscles of your face. Just keep relaxing your whole body like that for a while. And as you relax more and more, imagine your body becoming heavier and warmer. Imagine your body becoming pleasantly heavier. Imagine sinking deeper and deeper and deeper as you relax more and more and more. And imagine your body becoming warmer, pleasantly warmer as any signs of tension disappear. And as your relaxation grows, imagine sinking deeper and deeper and deeper into a state of perfect relaxation. In a state of perfect relaxation, you should feel unwilling to move a single muscle in your body.

Now you can become twice as relaxed by breathing slowly and rhythmically. You become less aware of objects and movements around you. You are concentrating solely on becoming more and more relaxed as your body becomes pleasantly heavier and pleasantly warmer. Just continue relaxing like that. When you want to get up, count backwards from 5 to 1. You should then feel fine and refreshed, wide awake and perfectly relaxed.

Progressive relaxation 2: Quick relaxation

Settle back as comfortably as you can. And begin by slowing down your breathing so that your breathing becomes much more relaxed so that your body can begin to relax immediately.

Concentrate on where the tension is in your body and concentrate on letting that tension go. I want you to imagine pushing any tension from the top of your head down to your toes. Just imagine any signs of tension being pushed down your forehead, down your face. Push the tension down, down, onto your neck so that your face becomes relaxed. Study any signs of tension on your face and let them be pushed down and down. Allow your face to relax and, by pushing the tension down and down, your neck relaxes.

Allow your shoulders to slope down and get rid of any tension from those muscles and push that tension down onto your arms. And feel the relaxation spreading down from your face, down from your shoulders, the relaxation spreading into your arms. And imagine the relaxation spreading down your arms, pushing any tension in front of it, pushing the tension right out of your arms down to the hands and pushing the tension right out of your body, out through your fingertips. Concentrate on relaxing the arms fully and deeply. Imagine your shoulders to your fingertips now relaxed. Let your arms become more and more relaxed.

And push any signs of tension down your chest. Down your stomach, pushing the tension down your legs so that your chest relaxes and your stomach relaxes. Concentrate again on your breathing, allowing your breathing to slow down so that it is very comfortable and relaxing for you. And allow your body to become more and more relaxed. And push this tension further down your legs. Push this tension as far away from you as you can; down through your thighs, down through the calf muscles and right out of your body, through your toes. And concentrate again on the spread of relaxation. Just allow the relaxation to spread down through your legs so that your thighs, your calf muscles and your feet now become pleasantly relaxed. And once again, just imagine your body becoming more and more relaxed. Your breathing relaxes your body more and more as your muscles become more and more relaxed.

And imagine your body becoming pleasantly heavy, pleasantly warm. Allow your body to become more and more deeply relaxed. Look out for any remaining signs of tension in your body. Isolate the tension and then push it out of your body. Concentrate on relaxing the areas of your body where you find tension. And allow those feelings of tension to disappear and be replaced by very pleasant feelings of relaxation. And if there are any worries in your mind right now, let them disappear. Let them go. Allow your mind to become as relaxed as your body. Concentrate only on pleasant relaxation.

And allow these feelings of relaxation to develop and enjoy them. And as this quick relaxation ends, I want you to carry this feeling of relaxation with you. Don't let tension creep back into your body; don't let tension creep back into your mind. Concentrate on relaxation and take it with you, no matter what you do today. And, in your own time, as you count down from 5 to 1, you will feel perfectly relaxed, perfectly alert, very pleasantly calm.

Leaves in the stream

This exercise teaches you to stand back and observe your stressful thoughts rather than get caught up in them. Notice that thoughts are simply thoughts, passing streams of words that we don't need to react to; we can just notice them. Sit quietly, close your eyes and focus on your breathing. Then start to notice the thoughts that come into your mind.

In your imagination, put each thought you notice onto a leaf and watch it drift down a stream. There is no need to look for the thoughts or remain alert, waiting for them to appear. Just let them come and, as they do, place them on a leaf and let them float gently away. Your attention may wander and that's OK; that's what your mind does. As soon as your mind wanders, gently bring your focus back to the thoughts and place them on the leaves. And after a few moments, bring your attention back to your breathing and open your eyes and become aware of your surroundings again.

Body scan

Close your eyes and breathe gently through your nose. As you breathe in, you may be aware that the air feels quite cool. And as you breathe out it feels warmer. You don't need to change the rate or the rhythm of your breathing at all. You are simply watching the breath as you breathe in and out. Just pay attention to your breathing for a few moments.

Now turn your attention to your chest. What are you aware of as you gently breathe in and breathe out? Where do you feel the breath? In the upper part of the chest or the lower part? Which muscles are moving? Which bones are moving as you gently breathe in and breathe out? If you can, as you breathe out, begin to feel that you can release, relax and let go. So each time you breathe in and breathe out, you learn to release, relax and let go. So simply by breathing you can begin to feel more peaceful, calmer and more relaxed.

Turn your attention to your feet. What are you aware of in your feet at this particular moment? Any particular sensations in your toes? Tingling? Numbness? Whether your feet feel hot or cold? Just think about how your feet are feeling. Now be aware of your legs, your skin, your muscles, the bones of your lower legs, knees, thighs. Just pay attention to what you are aware of in your feet and legs at this particular moment. And if you can, try to imagine that each breath is flowing through your legs, releasing, relaxing and letting go. So as you breathe in and breathe out, the breath flows away through your legs, and out through the tips of your toes, releasing, relaxing and letting go. And feel yourself relaxing and feeling at peace.

Turn your attention now to your hands. What are you aware of at this particular moment in your hands? The sensations in your fingertips, the palms of your hands, the back of your hands? Whatever the sensations may be, you are just paying attention and being aware of them.

Be aware now of your arms and shoulders – the skin, the bones, be aware of any tension, any tightness, any discomfort. You are simply noting it and being aware of it. And, as before, I'd like you to breathe in and, as you breathe out, feel as if the breath is flowing through your arms, releasing, relaxing and letting go. Just feel the breath flow away through your fingertips. You may be aware that your mind begins to wander; that you begin to think of other things. Don't worry about this, simply be aware of what is happening and then gently return your mind to listening to my voice and being aware of your breath each time you breathe in and breathe out. Release, relax and let go.

Now turn your attention to your face. What are you aware of in the muscles of your forehead, your eyes, your jaw, your mouth? Any tightness? Any tension? As before, you are going to breathe in, and as you breathe out you are going to release, relax and let go any tension in the muscles of your face. It is almost as if the breath is flowing through your face; through the muscles of your forehead, eyes, jaw. Releasing, relaxing and letting go.

Turn your attention to your head: the muscles on the top of your head, the back of your head, your neck and all the way down your spine. What is your awareness at this particular moment? Any tightness? Any tension? Any discomfort? And as before, you are going to breathe in, and as you breathe out the breath is going to flow over the top of your head, down the back of your head, all the way down your spine. Relaxing, releasing and letting go. Simply by the act of breathing, you can learn to relax, release and let go.

Now turn your attention back to your chest. You may be aware that you are breathing a little slower, a little deeper. If you can, I'd like you to imagine that you are able to breathe in and out of your tummy; as if your breathing is dropping even lower and you are breathing in through the centre of your tummy. And, as you breathe out, the breath simply flows away through the tips of your toes, through the tips of your fingers, the top of your head and the bottom of your spine. Releasing, relaxing and letting go. And feel yourself relaxing and feeling at peace. As your body learns to relax, you can learn the skills of relaxing your mind. You can become aware of how thoughts can dart into the mind and connect with emotions like fear or sadness or frustration. But you have no need to follow the thoughts into these emotions. You can just let the thoughts float away like leaves in a stream.

And you return your awareness to your breathing in the centre of your tummy and, to help your mind relax, I'd like you to think of somewhere calm, peaceful; perhaps somewhere you have been to recently or a long time ago. Somewhere you have been to in reality or somewhere you would like to go. And I would like you, in your imagination, to go to that place and rest there. I'd like you to settle into that peaceful place and imagine you are moving effortlessly and moving easily towards somewhere pleasant where you are going to rest for a few moments. As you move effortlessly and move easily through the scene, you may be aware of sounds; you may be aware of scents or fragrances that help you to feel calm or peaceful. There may be something you can reach out and touch. And think how that feels under your fingertips and how that sense of touch helps you feel. So calm, so peaceful. And as you settle in that peaceful place and rest there for a few moments, calm and safe, you look around you at the colours, and the light and the shade, what you can smell, what you can hear, what you can touch. And all these sensations help you feel more calm, more peaceful, more relaxed. And you become more aware of how comfortable your body has become and how restful your mind has become. And the more you practise this relaxation, the more skilful you will become at returning to these thoughts and feelings of calmness and peacefulness wherever and whenever you need to simply by the act of breathing and, as we reach the end, you can either open your eyes, feeling restored and refreshed, ready and able to do whatever you need to do, or, if you want, you can drift into a peaceful, refreshing sleep as this relaxation now ends.

Appendix 2

Additional resources

Video

The World Health Organisation has two videos based on the excellent books by Matthew Johnstone: 'I had a black dog: his name was depression' and 'Living with a black dog'.
www.youtube.com/watch?v=XiCrniLQGYc
www.youtube.com/watch?v=2VRRx7Mtep8

The books (under the same titles) are also available.

Websites

www.nhs.uk
www.mind.org.uk
www.getselfhelp.co.uk

Phone numbers

NHS non-emergency helpline 111 (England and Scotland), or 0845 46 47 (Wales). Note: Northern Ireland does not currently offer this service.
Samaritans (UK and ROI) 116 123

Online relaxation and mindfulness

www.stresscontrolaudio.com

Index